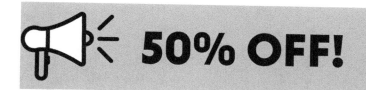 **50% OFF!**

MW00843816

MEDICAL-SURGICAL NURSE ONLINE TEST PREP COURSE

We consider it an honor and a privilege that you chose our Medical-Surgical Nurse Study Guide. As a way of showing our appreciation and to help us better serve you, we have partnered with Mometrix Test Preparation to offer you 50% off their online Medical-Surgical Nurse Prep Course.

Mometrix has structured their online course to perfectly complement your printed study guide. Many Medical-Surgical Nurse courses are needlessly expensive and don't deliver enough value. With their course, you get access to the best Medical-Surgical Nurse prep material, and you only pay half price.

WHAT'S IN THE MEDICAL-SURGICAL NURSE TEST PREP COURSE?

- ✓ **Medical-Surgical Nurse Study Guide**: Get access to content that complements your study guide.

- ✓ **Progress Tracker**: Their customized course allows you to check off content you have studied or feel confident with.

- ✓ **1,050+ Practice Questions**: With 1,050+ practice questions and lesson reviews, you can test yourself again and again to build confidence.

- ✓ **Medical-Surgical Nurse Flashcards**: Their course includes a flashcard mode consisting of over 350 content cards to help you study.

TO RECEIVE THIS DISCOUNT, VISIT THE WEBSITE AT

link.mometrix.com/medsurg

USE THE DISCOUNT CODE:
STARTSTUDYING

SCAN HERE

IF YOU HAVE ANY QUESTIONS OR CONCERNS, PLEASE CONTACT MOMETRIX AT SUPPORT@MOMETRIX.COM

Mometrix
ONLINE COURSES

Free DVD **FREE** Free DVD

Essential Test Tips Video from Trivium Test Prep

Dear Customer,

Thank you for purchasing from Trivium Test Prep! Whether you're looking to join the military, get into college, or advance your career, we're honored to be a part of your journey.

To show our appreciation (and to help you relieve a little of that test-prep stress), we're offering a **FREE** *Medical Surgical Nurse Essential Test Tips* **Video** by Trivium Test Prep. Our video includes 35 test preparation strategies that will help keep you calm and collected before and during your big exam. All we ask is that you email us your feedback and describe your experience with our product. Amazing, awful, or just so-so: we want to hear what you have to say!

To receive your **FREE** *Medical Surgical Nurse Essential Test Tips* **Video**, please email us at 5star@ triviumtestprep.com. Include "Free 5 Star" in the subject line and the following information in your email:

   1. The title of the product you purchased.

   2. Your rating from 1 – 5 (with 5 being the best).

   3. Your feedback about the product, including how our materials helped you meet your goals and ways in which we can improve our products.

   4. Your full name and shipping address so we can send your **FREE** *Medical Surgical Nurse Essential Test Tips* **Video**.

If you have any questions or concerns, please feel free to contact us directly at 5star@triviumtestprep.com.

Thank you, and good luck with your studies!

Med Surg Certification Review Book

2 Practice Tests and CMSRN Exam Study Guide for Medical Surgical Nursing Prep

Jeremy Downs

TABLE OF CONTENTS

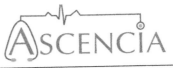

Patient/Care Management

Patient Safety

Patient Safety Protocols

Skin Integrity

Patients with compromised skin integrity are at risk for pressure injuries, incontinence-associated dermatitis, medical-device pressure injuries, and skin tears. Vulnerability can be due to several risk factors. Advanced age may lead to fragile skin because of reduced elasticity, poor hydration, and a thinning subcutaneous layer. Other medical conditions may affect circulation, cognition, or sensory perception. Limited mobility, urinary and fecal incontinence, and moisture from other bodily fluids negatively impact the skin barrier. Malnutrition because of insufficient hydration, protein, vitamins and minerals, and calorie intake impedes wound healing. Wearable medical devices (e.g., nasogastric tubes, urinary catheters, and oxygen tubing) may cause skin breakdown due to the device material, tape used for reinforcement, and constant or excess pressure. Skin injuries can lead to discomfort, increased risk of infection, increased length of stay, and increased risk of morbidity and mortality.

Evidence-based skin bundles can decrease patient harm. Skin assessment and intervention protocols and procedures vary according to facility. A complete and comprehensive skin assessment is performed during the initial patient admission, at least once during the shift, and more frequently as needed. Skin findings are described and documented in the patient's medical record. A pressure injury risk assessment tool, like the Braden scale, takes into consideration the patient's skin condition, mobility, and nutrition. The tool identifies high-risk patients and guides decision-making to protect the skin.

Purposeful rounding is a strategy the nurse can implement to prevent pressure injuries and skin breakdown. Basic hygiene, managing moisture, regular toileting or incontinence care, and linen changes when soiled aim to keep the skin clean and dry. Ongoing assessment, monitoring, and care of devices enable the nurse to identify and prevent medical device-related pressure injuries. Support surfaces (i.e., limb protectors, air-filled overlays, and low air-loss beds) offload and redistribute pressure. Patients should also be assisted with mobility that is appropriate for the patient at least every two hours. Ambulation, range of motion, turning, and repositioning promote circulation to protect the skin. Providing adequate hydration and nutrition prevents malnourishment. Skin care products (i.e., skin barriers) are used to promote healing and maintain skin integrity. Patients deemed at high risk for skin breakdown may require additional support through a wound care professional and/or nutritionist consult.

Infection

Risk factors for infection include age, multiple comorbidities, malnutrition, immunosuppression, hospitalization, prolonged hospital length of stay, invasive procedures, mechanical ventilation, and indwelling medical devices. For example, a hospitalized older adult patient with multiple comorbidities of diabetes, high blood pressure, and morbid obesity is at a higher risk of infection.

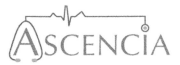

Infection prevention bundles may vary between facilities. These evidenced-based interventions promote consistency among nursing care delivery and good patient outcomes. Common infection prevention bundles reduce catheter-associated urinary tract infections (CAUTI), central line-associated bloodstream infection (CLABSI), ventilator-associated pneumonia (VAP), and surgical site infections (SSI).

An indwelling urinary catheter in place for two or more calendar days puts the patient at risk for developing a CAUTI. The appropriateness of the catheter must be considered prior to placement. After insertion, the nurse assesses the necessity during every shift and discontinues the device as soon as it is no longer required. Other measures to prevent infection are using hand hygiene prior to insertion, employing aseptic technique, keeping the tubing free from kinks, maintaining the collection bag below the level of the bladder, and washing the insertion site with soap and water daily and when needed.

To decrease harm from a CLABSI, the device should also be evaluated for necessity and discontinued as soon as possible. Femoral access is avoided when possible. A designated trained licensed staff member inserts the central line, typically using a checklist. Infection control measures include hand hygiene and maximal sterile barrier precautions, skin preparation with chlorhexidine, ultrasound-guided placement, and use of a securement device. Maintenance includes changing the dressing per facility protocol and when visibly soiled or loose. Catheter hubs, needleless connections, and injection ports are disinfected using port protectors and proper cleaning (i.e., scrubbing the hub) prior to line access.

Patients who require mechanical ventilation as a result of respiratory failure are at risk for VAP, which can develop after forty-eight hours of intubation. The necessity of the device is first evaluated and alternative devices (e.g., continuous positive airway pressure) are attempted first. Decreasing the ventilation time and weaning the patient as soon as possible are methods to prevent infection. Commonly used bundles are elevating the head of bed between thirty to forty-five degrees, daily sedation interruptions to avoid oversedation, meticulous oral care, subglottic secretion drainage, changing the ventilator circuit when visibly soiled or malfunctioning, and DVT prophylaxis. Patients who receive enteral nutrition via nasogastric tube may experience a higher risk of gastroesophageal reflux (GER), which can consequently lead to VAP.

The prevention of SSIs can occur through bathing the body with an antiseptic agent, administering antibiotic prophylaxis when indicated, proper skin preparation by the surgical team, monitoring blood glucose with a desired level less than 200 mg/dL, and maintaining the patient's core body temperature before and after surgery.

Falls

Patient falls are a large culprit of injury and affect functional status, mobility, morbidity, and mortality. Patients are at risk of falling in the healthcare setting due to present medical conditions, medications, or the general patient environment. Fall risk assessments, such as the Morse Fall Scale, seek to identify high risk factors on admission and every shift. A recent history of falling, older age, altered mental status or cognitive issues, certain medications, use of assistive devices, altered mobility, and certain medical diagnoses (e.g., orthopedic surgery, delirium, hypotension) should be assessed for each patient. Other factors may be related to physical disabilities, vision and hearing impairments, pain, and emotional states. Environmental hazards may include clutter, slippery surfaces, and scatter rugs.

Medications can be a significant contributing factor. Cardiac medication may decrease blood pressure or heart rate, leading to dizziness or syncope. Diuretics may create urinary urgency and frequent ambulation to the toilet. Opioids, benzodiazepines, and antipsychotics may lead to drowsiness, impaired

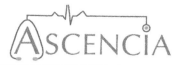

gait, cognitive changes, or orthostatic hypotension. If intravenous fluids are given, patients must walk with an IV pole, a piece of equipment that could create a fall hazard.

In addition to fall risk assessments, interventions can lessen potential fall hazards. Fall risk bundles vary across facilities. One example is Fall TIPS (Tailoring Intervention for Patient Safety), a patient-centered fall prevention toolkit. Individualized visual signage includes patient education as well as reminders for interventions such as mobility assistance, assistive devices, toileting schedule, and bed alarm (within facility protocol). Other common interventions include visual cues that include a color-specific fall alert, identification wristband or bracelet charm, door signs, and chair alarms (within facility protocol). Patients exhibiting significant altered cognition may have room placement closer to the nursing station, increased checks, and/or use of a telesitter or in-person sitter.

Communicating about patients who are at risk for falling is an essential part of nursing practice. Safety huddles alert all staff of patients who are most vulnerable. Bedside handoff can provide a visual safety check for the incoming nurse. Purposeful rounding addresses anticipated needs, including assistance with repositioning, pain relief, personal needs like toileting or incontinence care, and placement of necessary items. Additionally, the room is checked to confirm that the nursing call light is within reach, bed/chair alarms are in place (within facility protocol), and the bed is in a low and locked position. Following a patient fall, a huddle may be conducted by staff members to identify any potential causes and work to prevent future falls.

Restraints

Restraints are used for patients who exhibit aggressive behavior changes when other alternatives (e.g., toileting, de-escalation) have been exhausted and the patient is at a high risk for self-harm or harming another person. A physician assesses the patient in person within a specified timeframe according to state and facility regulations. An order must be present in the medical record. The nurse thoroughly documents the restraint reason, assessment, and interventions that are performed while the patient is restrained. Restraints are removed as soon as clinically indicated to support patient autonomy and dignity. Although used to address behavior, restraints may contribute to harm or injury. Ramifications of restraint use are cognitive changes, hospital-acquired pressure injuries, deconditioning, and agitation.

Two types of restraints in the medical-surgical setting are physical and chemical restraints. Approved physical restraints are mechanical devices that are applied in order to limit range of motion and prevent the patient from moving freely. The nurse should keep in mind that any material that restricts the patient's freedom of movement, including the use of all four side rails, tucking sheets tightly into the bed, and holding the patient in a way that they cannot move freely, is a form of restraint. Restraints are applied according to the current patient behavior and prudent medical provider involvement. Like physical restraints, chemical restraints are ONLY applied with the direct consultation and approval from the licensed physician with a written order.

Restraint assessments vary according to facility and depend upon state guidelines. When physical restraints are used, frequent monitoring is required in order to prevent injury. The patient is evaluated at a specified time interval by the nurse according to institutional policy. Assessment of skin and circulation is performed as well as assessing for earliest discontinuation of any restraints. Nursing interventions include active range of motion, ensuring adequate hydration and nutrition, and providing toileting.

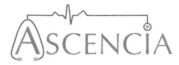

Suicide/Mental Wellness

Nurses play a pivotal role in the prevention of suicide when caring for a vulnerable patient. A suicide risk assessment includes identifying patient risk factors. A medical, emotional, and behavioral screening should be conducted on all patients. The patient may have a history of trauma, recent losses, or previous suicide attempts. The patient may have emotional symptoms, such as feeling isolated, lonely, or hopeless, or physical symptoms, such as chronic pain. Other factors include a mental health disorder, substance use, a newly diagnosed medical condition, chronic illness, recent loss, and family history.

Bundles of care may differ across facilities, and interventions are defined by organizational policy and procedure. One example of a screening tool is the Columbia-Suicide Severity Rating Scale (C-SSRS). The nurse uses specific yes or no queries. The screening includes questions that inquire whether the patient actively wishes to be dead, has active suicidal thoughts, and has active suicidal ideation with or without a plan to act. Other queries inquire about the intensity of the suicidal ideation, including frequency, duration, anything that deters the patient from acting on suicidal thoughts. Specific questions about any attempts are also asked. Documentation of the risk assessment should occur in the medical record.

Early recognition and intervention are key aspects of keeping patients from harming themselves. The nurse communicates with the patient in a nonjudgmental manner to create a trusting relationship. Upon identification of an active suicide risk, a patient-specific safety plan is created. An environmental hazard checklist may be used to ensure that the room is as safe as possible, removing sharp objects, extra linen, and objects that are not needed. The collaboration of the healthcare team is important to the support of the patient. The patient requires continuous monitoring by a trained staffed member. A psychiatric healthcare provider evaluates the patient to determine immediate needs. Discharge planning includes community support information, including a crisis hotline and support group information, along with any follow-up referrals or appointments.

Factors in Patient and Nurse Safety

Environmental

Environmental safety is a significant component of high-quality patient outcomes. Consider the patient admitted with cognitive disabilities. Clinical judgment must be used to decrease stimuli, such as lighting and noise. Hospital beds are placed in the lowest and locked position with appropriate side rails in place. Electrical cords and wires are situated away to prevent a possible fall.

The medical-surgical nurse plays a central role in other safety measures, including infection protocols, waste management, and emergency equipment. Infection control measures such as hand hygiene, washing down equipment, and implementing necessary infection control precautions prevent the spread of infectious organisms. Linens may be a reservoir for pathogens due to contaminated body fluids and are placed in designated containers to prevent the transfer of microorganisms. Determining and eliminating resources that do not have value is an essential part of waste management. For example, the prudent use of linens eliminates the storage of unneeded supplies in patient rooms.

Emergency equipment contents must be reviewed, verified, and maintained according to institutional policy and procedure. The code cart, which contains medication, supplies, and other emergency items, is kept ready for use. Supplies are intact without expired dates. Oxygen tanks are full. Correct sizes of equipment are accessible. If elements are missing, then the emergency response could result in an error, a delay in care, and a poor patient outcome.

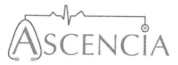

Medication management is another cornerstone of patient safety. Clean and aseptic technique in medication preparation and administration prevents infection. Proper medication disposal is a component of waste management designed to avoid environmental harm, such as contamination of a water source. Not disposing of controlled substances, such as opioids, in proper receptacles may cause the potential for misuse or diversion.

Transitions in care are a risk for patient safety. The nurse provides the patient with education regarding prescribed home medications including proper disposal, side effects, and potential interactions. If safety is a concern, the patient may require other discharge needs such as modifications to the home environment. Improved lighting, eliminating falling hazards (e.g., throw rugs or clutter), and installation of grab bars can increase general home safety. The home may need to be assessed for fire and electrical safety, carbon monoxide exposure, and water quality as well.

Finally, a healthy work environment and a supportive organizational culture contributes to safety among nurses. Components of a supportive organizational culture include facilitating a zero-tolerance policy for violence, encouraging nursing staff to report problems without fear of retaliation, and ensuring access to safety equipment. Sufficient staffing is also crucial for a healthy work environment because it reduces turnover, increases nursing satisfaction, and decreases the potential risk for error and injury.

Skill-Related

Human error may come at a great cost to patient well-being. It also contributes to patient morbidity and mortality. Reflect on the patient admitted to a medical-surgical unit who requires a urinary catheter. Three days following insertion, the patient develops a fever, lethargy, and cloudy urine. A urine culture reveals a urinary tract infection. The patient now requires IV antibiotics and must remain in the hospital longer than anticipated due to the nosocomial infection. The catheter-acquired urinary tract infection (CAUTI) could have been prevented with aseptic insertion technique, diligent care of the device, and frequent evaluation of catheter necessity.

Staff education, policies, and procedures aim to protect all stakeholders. Medical harm has implications for both the nurse and the patient. For example, not implementing safe patient handling measures could negatively affect the patient's comfort and safety as well as result in staff injury. Good lifting and transferring techniques, along with the correct use of equipment (i.e., mechanical lifts and transfer devices) can help prevent injuries. Medication errors also encompass a large aspect of medical harm. Effective communication, proper patient identification, following the five medication rights, identifying abnormal diagnostic values, and carefully monitoring the patient are all important aspects of safe nursing practice.

Careful assessment skills and clinical judgment determine the nursing diagnosis for guiding care. The impact of overlooking basic care, assessment findings, outcomes to interventions, patient education, and/or discharge planning can be detrimental to the patient. For example, a lack of patient education could result in complications of their care, hindrances in discharge planning, and ineffective patient decision-making. Missed and delayed care impact patient satisfaction, the nurse-patient relationship, potential for readmission, length of stay, and patient outcomes.

Process-Related

Patient safety risk factors that are process-related include miscommunication, which plays a large role in human error. The nurse can feel rushed, misunderstand the received message, and/or have a poor working relationship. For example, if the nurse does not comprehend the medication order, the patient may receive the wrong dose. Lack of streamlined methods of communication may contribute to

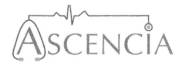

communication barriers. With multiple platforms of communication available, it is critical for the nurse to follow the organization's protocol for communication mediums and use all approved abbreviations for safe and effective communication.

Policies and procedures guide nursing practice and decision-making. Medication safety is one example. Organizations clearly define unacceptable abbreviations, outline the standardized time for medication administration, and create a process to report adverse events. Safety reports are submitted for follow up and investigation, with an outlined recommendation for an action plan. Procedures like infection prevention protocols are in place to mitigate safety risks. For example, for indwelling urinary catheters, protocols guide the initiation of precautionary measures as well as the discontinuation as soon as medically appropriate. These protocols streamline and standardize processes to reduce infectious disease.

Technology can be a cybersecurity risk that affects both patient privacy and confidentiality. Nurses play a pivotal role in protecting private patient information by not sharing unique passwords, avoiding opening attachments from unknown senders, and identifying strangers who should not be near computer devices or medical records. Downtime, whether planned or unplanned, can be an enormous disruption to patient care because most medical information is stored as an electronic record. As a result, nurses may become overwhelmed with decision-making and clinical judgment during the disruption in workflow. To prepare for downtime, the nurse must follow the organization's business continuity plan, which typically consists of maintaining up-to-date paper charts and paper documentation forms.

Human Factors

Other human factors play a role in compromising patient safety. Strategies to reduce error are implemented as organizational goals. While eliminating all errors is not feasible, the organizational culture is an essential part of error reduction. If the organizational climate does not support employee well-being, staff turnover and job dissatisfaction may increase. Maintaining sufficient staffing of nursing units and ensuring that staff input is valued contribute to a healthy environment. Otherwise, patients are at higher risk of negative outcomes, including infections, falls, and increased rates of mortality.

The nurse's own well-being can also contribute negatively to patient care. Consider the nurse who is fatigued and not making comprehensive clinical decisions. If nurses have not received an adequate break or feel depleted of energy, hungry, or dehydrated, mistakes may happen, resulting in a near-miss or patient harm. Emotional stress may preclude the nurse from communicating well with the patient or healthcare team. When nurses feel overwhelmed or rushed, they may neglect to perform a safety check of the patient before leaving the room. Bed alarms might be missed, which could lead to a patient falling. Failure to document significant clinical changes may lead to gaps in patient care and poor communication within the medical record.

Care Bundles

Nursing care bundles, checklists, and algorithms are evidence-based tools that are used to support patient safety and mitigate harm. A nursing care bundle uses several evidence-based interventions together to achieve a successful outcome for each patient. Checklists outline and document the steps involved in a certain high-risk procedure to ensure an item is not missed. An algorithm is a tool that guides evidence-based practice by providing a decision-tree to follow based on different scenarios.

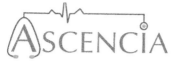

Patient Safety Culture

Nurse leaders have the ability to establish an organizational culture that promotes patient safety. Human error cannot be completely avoided. Nurses face certain obstacles when reporting errors such as being perceived as incompetent, dislike of criticism, and concern for retribution. Think about the nurse who continuously pulls the wrong IV fluid from the supply room. It would be easy to associate the error with incompetence, but upon further investigation, the nurse leader may come to realize that the storage room on his routine unit has the correct IV fluid stored in that same location. Knowing this, the nurse leader can have a simple training session with the employee and suggest to senior leadership the importance of consistency in the organization of the supply rooms. The potential for error can be lessened significantly by a system that prevents risk as much as possible.

Just Culture

Poor communication, including not reporting an issue that may cause the patient harm, impedes safe care. In a just culture, leaders encourage nurses to report errors and potential for harm without fear of retaliation. Barriers to safe practice should be identified and addressed instead of punishing those who commit errors. This culture empowers nurses to identify and discuss necessary changes to protect and advocate for the patient.

Near-Miss Reporting

Near-miss reporting contributes to a culture of patient safety. A near-miss event is described as an error that could have resulted in significant harm in a different circumstance or if the error had not been recognized. For example, the patient is reporting itchiness and would like a dose of hydroxyzine. The nurse retrieves the item from the medication dispensing system and notices that the drug is labeled hydralazine. She realizes the mistake and finds another tablet that is labeled properly. Her patient is not harmed. Speaking up and communicating issues that could cause serious injury or harm may prevent actual harm from occurring in the future.

Barriers to near-miss reporting include perceiving the issue as insignificant, time involved to report problems, and lack of follow-up by nursing leadership. Consider what would happen if the nurse did not have time to report the near-miss. Another nurse could take the medication without looking at the label and administer hydralazine instead of hydroxyzine. The patient could experience dizziness with a subsequent syncopal episode. Despite obstacles to reporting, being proactive and advocating for patient safety protect patients from harm.

The Occupational Safety and Health Administration (OSHA) advises that employees report all near-miss events. If organizational cultures do not support a just culture of speaking up, then opportunity to prevent injury or harm does not happen. Leadership responsibility encompasses quality improvement by identifying and decreasing risks. Methods that employers can use to encourage staff to share near-miss events are incorporating a policy, instilling education, allowing for reporting methods to be streamlined and comprehensible, establishing a non-punitive culture for near-miss reporting, and recognizing progress achieved.

Patient Safety Assessments and Reporting

Abuse and Neglect

The medical-surgical nurse is responsible for recognizing risk factors for abuse and neglect. Victims may experience physical, emotional, and/or sexual abuse. The most vulnerable populations exploited tend to

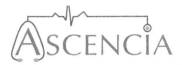

be those who are dependent on care by others, such as children, older adults, disabled people, homeless individuals, and those with debilitating chronic conditions. Pediatric and geriatric populations are among those with the highest risk. The nursing assessment is key to identifying signs and symptoms of abuse. This focused nursing assessment should include gathering medical history, documenting noticeable findings, observing interactions between the patient and caregivers, and promptly reporting any abuse.

Children may be abused by a parent, another caregiver, or a person with a close relationship to them. Physical abuse may result in physical impact with manifestations of unexplained skin conditions, like bruising caused by force or burns. Multiple bruises that are all in different stages of healing can also be a warning sign for potential abuse. The child may exhibit an abrasion or laceration. Bone fractures may also be noted. The child may be fearful or anxious around the abuser. Emotional abuse can occur when the abuser does not meet emotional needs of the child, which often negatively affects self-worth and can hinder development. For example, the abuser may verbally assault or withhold affection from the child. This can lead to certain habits (e.g., frequent picking at skin/scabs) or affect learning and development. Sexual abuse includes rape, molestation, or incest. The child may exhibit developmental regressions (e.g., bedwetting), have nightmares, frequently rebel, or have exaggerated mood swings. There may be physical signs of injury around the genitalia, such as bruising, pain, or torn underwear.

The older adult may be a victim of abuse due to dependency as a result of a medical condition, cognitive disorders, or lack of mobility. In addition to physical, emotional, and sexual abuse, the older adult may also be taken advantage of financially. Signs of physical abuse may be like those of the child. The older adult may also have unexplained bruising, lacerations, fractures, or burns. Examples of emotional harm are yelling at the senior adult, making false accusations, or engaging in humiliation. As a result, the senior may become forgetful, fearful, or withdrawn. Sexual abuse can be recognized by unexplained physical signs of injury around the genitalia, sexually transmitted diseases, or torn underwear.

Nurses are among the professionals mandated to report suspected incidents of abuse and neglect. Reporting is defined by state law and commonly extends to physicians, social workers, mental health professionals, teachers, child care providers, and law enforcement. The potential for penalties or charges exists if the nurse neglects to report a suspected or confirmed issue.

Human Trafficking

Human trafficking victims may exhibit similar signs as people who have experienced abuse. Victims may show signs of physical trauma, such as lacerations, scars, burns, bite marks, and bruising. With human trafficking for sex, patients may have sexually transmitted diseases, trauma to the vagina or rectum, urinary tract infections, or unwanted pregnancies. Furthermore, victims may appear malnourished, fatigued, and dehydrated. Other indicators may be noted from the individual accompanying the patient. The individual may insist on speaking for the patient or constantly supervising the patient. The victim may speak little English, be unaware of surroundings, act submissive with closed body language, and/or appear scared or anxious. Often the abuser controls the victim's identification documents and finances.

Because victims rarely speak out, blatant signs of human trafficking may be difficult to detect. Medical care may only be sought out if the trafficked victim is very sick. Often the patient will be accompanied by their controller. A careful assessment includes noting the physical signs of abuse, as well as asking prudent questions. Questions must be asked in privacy without the accompanied person. If a language barrier is evident, a translator approved by the agency/facility should be used. Asking open-ended questions gives the victim the opportunity to describe their situation. Because victims tend to exhibit shame surrounding their situation, the nurse's empathy can foster the nurse-patient relationship.

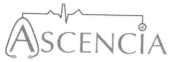

The requirements for reporting human trafficking can depend on the state. If the patient is a minor, the nurse is a mandated reporter of abuse. Each institution has a policy outlining the protocol to report human trafficking, and the nurse should be prepared to properly screen, provide care, and provide emotional support for these patients based on these policies and procedures. The National Human Trafficking Resource Center hotline can be provided to victims for additional support and resources.

Elopement

Patient elopement occurs when a patient dependent on care leaves the healthcare setting without permission or knowledge of the nursing staff and poses a risk of harm to themselves or other people. Reflect upon the patient with a history of mild dementia. The new environment causes an increase in confusion and the patient leaves with the objective of returning home. Next, consider the patient with hepatic encephalopathy who initially is confused and decides to leave without notifying the nurse.

Risk factors for elopement include cognitive impairment, as seen with patients who have dementia, delirium, traumatic brain injury, or medication-related changes. The patient may appear agitated or restless, express desire to leave or go home, have recently experienced changes in his environment or routine, and have recent medication changes. Often the patient is mobile and may have a history of wandering. The patient is set on leaving the healthcare facility without discussion with the staff. Patients who elope are at risk of harm, or even death, from injury, accidents, or inclement weather.

Nursing interventions for patients at risk for elopement include performing frequent nursing checks, using a bed or chair alarm (within facility policy, as this can be considered a restraint), providing close observation (i.e., placing the patient in a room right next to the nurses' station), encouraging the presence of family, and providing diversional activities. Addressing basic care needs, such as frequent toileting, offering food or drink, and assisting with mobility are also important.

Social Determinants

The complexity of social determinants for each individual patient plays a major role in patient safety. When caring for patients with complex needs, the nurse must remain empathetic and nonjudgmental. Inadequate resources such as unsafe housing, lack of transportation, and limited access to clean water or healthy food interfere with patient safety. Risk factors include people who are living in rural areas or inner cities and individuals who are impoverished, less educated, and isolated from human services.

Older residences may contain lead, which can adversely affect health. For example, lead exposure among children may lead to neurotoxicity, allergy flare-ups, and asthma exacerbation. Additionally, people may not have the necessary utilities, such as heat or electricity. The inability to access consistent transportation can influence well-being, as it can interfere with grocery shopping, traveling to healthcare appointments, or picking up medications. There may be a lower supply of fresh produce and a higher number of fast-food restaurants. Risky behaviors, like alcohol consumption, smoking, and illicit drug use, can negatively affect a patient's health. Community violence may be prevalent as a result of gun-related incidences or gang violence. There may also be inadequate safe spaces for community gatherings or exercising. Discharge planning can help ensure that patients receive appropriate follow-up care with resources provided for overcoming the social determinants in place (e.g., meal delivery services or community transportation resources)

Risk Assessment Methods

Risk assessment methods identify patients at high risk for adverse events as a result of their medical care. Proactive interventions can keep the patient free from injury. Risk assessments contribute to a

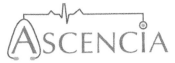

culture of safety through mitigating falls, hospital-acquired infections, postoperative complications, and medical error. Evidence-based practices like safety huddles are used so the staff can discuss anticipated problems and communicate high risk patients, environmental concerns, and other issues. Huddles promote shared understanding, teamwork, and staff satisfaction.

Rounding is used to meet patient needs, address issues, and promote safe patient care practices. Examples include purposeful or hourly rounding, discharge planning rounds, and nurse leader rounds. Purposeful rounding means that the patient is seen at regular intervals. The nurse intentionally addresses pain, toileting, positioning, comfort, and environmental safety. When the nurse addresses needs before they arise, injuries can be prevented.

Two methods to evaluate contributing factors of harm are a Root Cause Analysis (RCA) and Failure Mode and Effects Analysis (FMEA). An RCA is a quality improvement method that seeks to identify the root causes of an issue after harm or a breakdown in care occurs. The interprofessional team examines the data, evaluates the root causes, and identifies improvements. Communication failure, environmental problems, and staffing issues may play a role. For example, consider the patient who falls during a bed-to-chair transfer using a transfer device. The RCA may discover that there was not sufficient training and education on the transfer device. The RCA is a reactive method for improving patient care.

An FMEA analyzes potential events or problems that could lead to harm due to existing conditions or new changes. For example, changes are set to take place using a different medical device to prevent tubing misconnections. The staff may perform an FMEA to determine the actual risk and potential harm of tubing misconnections, the products affected, the stakeholders involved, and the education required. The FMEA is a proactive method for improving safe patient care. Emergency Preparedness plans for public health threats, such as natural disasters, bioterrorism emergencies, and pandemics. Value Analysis focuses on the supply chain and analyzes, for instance, the lowest cost products for the highest effectiveness.

Infection Prevention

Universal and Transmission-Based Precautions

Universal Precautions

Universal precautions are standardized measures implemented to protect healthcare workers from infectious diseases related to bloodborne pathogens. Examples of bloodborne pathogens include human immunodeficiency virus (HIV), hepatitis B, and hepatitis C. Exposure can result from contact with infectious fluids via open wounds, splashes of infectious fluids onto mucous membranes, or the improper handling of used equipment (e.g., accidental needle stick after use). A key point of universal precautions is the consistent use of these practices regardless of the patient's health status. Because the knowledge of infection transmission has evolved, so has the concept of universal standards. Standard precautions encompass all the universal precautions, but focus on the assumption that all bodily fluids may transmit infection.

Hand hygiene, personal protective equipment (PPE), sharps safety, and proper management of unclean equipment are all examples of universal precautions. Hand hygiene is a key component of infection control. Properly rubbing hands with an alcohol-based hand sanitizer or washing hands with soap and water should be performed on a routine basis. Hand hygiene is completed before and after patient

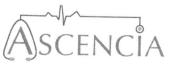

contact, before and after glove use, and when hands are visibly soiled. Soap and water are advised when hands are visibly soiled and for specific patient symptoms (e.g., frequent diarrhea with suspicion of *C. diff*).

PPE is worn to protect the nurse from possible exposure of infectious pathogens by body secretions and splashes. Gloves are applied prior to contact with anticipated body fluid or broken skin. A gown safeguards the skin and clothes from body fluids during patient care activities. A mask and eye protection, including goggles or a face shield, prevents splashes from fluids or secretions onto the nurse's face.

The transmission of organisms can also occur through sharp objects, such as needles. Safe practices consist of using a proper technique when handling the sharp, and engaging the safety gauge upon completion of use. Sharps are disposed of immediately in a designated waste container. Training and education should be received by the nurse prior to using an unfamiliar device in order to decrease the risk of injury.

The nurse will regularly participate in the handling of contaminated equipment. Patient-specific equipment must be cleaned between uses with facility-defined disinfecting agents. Soiled linen is placed in a designated laundry bin. Dirty patient equipment is stored in a separate location from clean supplies. The nurse also follows organizational policies and procedures for the disposal of biohazard waste.

Transmission-Based Precautions

Transmission-based precautions require additional protection beyond standard precautions. The three major categories of transmission are contact, droplet, and airborne. A combination may be used if needed. For example, airborne and contact precautions are required for chicken pox, which is caused by the varicella-zoster virus. Additional considerations for the nurse caring for a patient on transmission-based precautions include single room patient assignment, separate patient equipment (or disposable equipment if available), and additional room environment disinfection.

Infection Control Practices and Standards

Contact Precautions

Contact precautions are used when the pathogen is spread through contact with the patient's skin or body secretions or surfaces in the patient environment. Pathogens may be present on the skin or in bodily fluids. Examples include *Staphylococcus aureus*, group A streptococcus (droplet precautions are also required for the first twenty-four hours of treatment), and acute diarrhea. Infection or colonization with multidrug-resistant bacteria also frequently warrants these precautions, like methicillin-resistant *Staphylococcus aureus* (MRSA), vancomycin-resistant enterococci (VRE), and *Clostridium difficile* (C. diff). Hand hygiene is performed prior to entering and upon exiting the patient room.

Gloves and gowns are worn with contact precautions to prevent the spread of the infectious organism. Don PPE by fully fastening the gown and ensuring that the arms and trunk are covered. Next, apply gloves with the opening pulled over the gown wrists. After patient contact, the outside of the gloves and front of the gown and sleeves are considered the most contaminated. Doff PPE by removing the dirty gloves first. The outside of one glove is touched with the opposite hand, pulled off, and kept in the gloved hand. Then the glove-free fingers are inserted underneath the other glove for removal. The glove is pulled away over the first glove. Once the gloves are discarded, the gown is unfastened. The fingers are inserted on the inside of the neck region (non-contaminated side) and then pulled away, rolling from the inside.

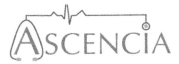

Droplet Precautions

Droplet precautions are indicated when the pathogen is transmitted through oral or nasal secretions when talking, coughing, or sneezing. The droplets extend approximately three to six feet from the patient before falling. For example, these precautions are indicated for patients diagnosed with *Neisseria meningitidis* (*Meningococcus*), influenza, adenovirus, and respiratory syncytial virus (RSV). Hand hygiene is performed when entering and upon exiting the patient room.

Droplet precautions include face and eye coverings for the eyes, nose, and mouth. A mask is worn with either goggles or a face shield. The mask is donned by placing the elastic over the ears, then ensuring that the mask is secure over the bridge of the nose and below the chin. The goggles or face shield is then placed accordingly. The outside of the goggles and face shield, as well as the front of the mask is considered the most contaminated. To remove, the nurse lifts the goggle ear pieces or the head securement of the face shield away from the head. The equipment is placed in the appropriate waste receptacle or disinfected per protocol. Then the mask is removed by placing the fingers under the elastic ear pieces and pulling away from the face. The mask can then be discarded. If contact precautions are also required, the donning sequence would be gown, mask, goggles or face shield, and gloves. The doffing procedure would be gloves, goggles or face shield, gown, and mask.

Airborne Precautions

Airborne precautions are used when a patient has a known or suspected infection capable of being transmitted through the air through aerosolized particles. The patient is placed in an airborne infection isolation (AII) room, which is maintained at a negative pressure. The system uses negative pressure to allow the influx of outside air into the room while either dispersing the contaminated air directly outdoors (where it will be immediately diluted) or passing the contaminated air through a HEPA filter prior to it circulating back to the general population. Examples of airborne infections include tuberculosis, measles, and severe acute respiratory syndrome virus (SARS-CoV). Contact precautions are frequently implemented with airborne precautions. PPE is often donned and doffed in an anteroom, while the patient door is kept closed until the nurse is ready to enter or exit the patient room.

Airborne precautions require a fit-tested N-95 mask or higher-level respirator (i.e., powered air-purifying respirator). Hand hygiene is performed, then the equipment is placed prior to entering the isolation room. The mask or respirator should be well-fitting. After the nurse has entered the patient room, the front of the mask or respirator is considered the most contaminated part of the equipment. To remove the mask, the nurse holds the elastic and pulls the mask away from the face without handling the front. The respirator is doffed by holding the bottom and pulling away from the head. If other PPE is required, the donning procedure would be: gown, mask or respirator, goggles or face shield (if no helmet), and gloves. The sequence for doffing is: gloves, goggles or face shield, gown, and mask or respirator. Hand hygiene is completed when exiting the patient room.

Current Evidence-Based Practice for Infection Control and Prevention Procedures

Evidence-based practice promotes a standardized approach to nursing care that incorporates scientific-based outcomes. Instead of following outdated concepts, the nurse practices according to up-to-date knowledge to guide decisions in support of excellent patient outcomes. The goal of evidence-based practice is to improve patient outcomes, reduce harm, and decrease financial burden. One example is oral care. Historically, oral care has been regarded as a basic hygiene need. Newer research shows data

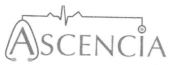

that increased oral care is an effective infection control measure among hospitalized patients to reduce hospital-acquired pneumonia, one of the most prominent hospital-acquired infections. The adoption of an evidenced-based nurse-driven protocol evaluates the type of oral care device, according to the level of assistance required by the patient, oral care procedure, and frequency. By reducing hospital-acquired pneumonia, the patient avoids a hospital-acquired infection, potential harm, and financial burden from extended hospital stays and additional treatments.

Universal precautions are well established to protect healthcare workers from blood-borne pathogens. Since the adoption of universal precautions set forth by the Occupational Health and Safety Administration (OSHA), infectious agents were noted to also occur by way of different transmission modes, like respiratory droplets. The Centers for Disease Control and Prevention (CDC) advises standard precautions for all patient care activities to protect healthcare workers and prevent infection transmission among patients. Although the concepts are similar, they are distinct from one another. Universal precautions now frequently include standard precautions.

Standard precautions incorporate basic infection control measures for every patient. These measures are widely discussed in nursing literature and by professional nursing bodies: hand hygiene, cough etiquette, sharps safety, environmental services, and asepsis. Cough etiquette is encouraged among all patients, visitors, and staff. Frequently, signage is posted in institutions for education indicating that coughing or sneezing should occur into the elbow to prevent hand contamination and followed by hand hygiene. Environmental services play a major role in the disinfecting of the patient environment and reusable equipment. Aseptic technique maintains a well-defined separation of equipment from clean and dirty. The nurse communicates any transmission precautions for appropriate cleaning.

Antimicrobial Stewardship

The widespread use and overuse of antimicrobial therapy has led to multidrug-resistant organisms (MDRO). These bacteria are not susceptible to certain antimicrobial treatments (e.g., vancomycin-resistant *enterococcus* (VRE) and methicillin-resistant *staphylococcus aureus* (MRSA)). Antimicrobial stewardship is the judicious prescribing and use of antimicrobials so that their effectiveness can be achieved while resistance is lessened. Thoughtful practice includes using narrow-spectrum drugs instead of broad-spectrum whenever possible, choosing the most appropriate dose, and selecting a reasonable duration. Among the stakeholders of physicians, pharmacists, and infection control staff, nurses play a pivotal role in antimicrobial stewardship practices.

At the time of admission, the nurse obtains the patient's medical history, assists with medication reconciliation, and reviews allergies. The patient's history may identify factors that can lead to hospital-acquired infections with subsequent antimicrobial administration. These include increased age, complex health conditions, and compromised immunity. Upon medication review, unnecessary antimicrobial prescriptions can be discovered and eliminated if needed. Patient allergies are differentiated between a true allergy and milder side effects. Although both are undesired outcomes, side effects (e.g., gastrointestinal symptoms, headache, vertigo) can be managed. More serious adverse events (e.g., anaphylaxis, hepatotoxicity, nephrotoxicity) can be life-threatening. The nurse must use clinical judgment in discerning these patient responses. Patients identified with a true allergy may require ordering of broad-spectrum antimicrobials, which can contribute to *C. diff* or an MDRO.

The nurse is considered a gatekeeper in preventing harm before a medication is administered. Prior to administration, the nurse engages in tasks that prompt the ordering of antimicrobial therapy. Often the collection of specimens, including urine, feces, sputum, and wound cultures, are nursing interventions performed when an infection is suspected. Clean and aseptic techniques are required so that the

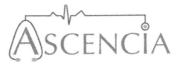

cultures are not contaminated. When reviewing the medication order and addressing concerns with the healthcare provider, the nurse advocates for the patient to receive the proper dose. Clinical progress and response to the treatment are essential to relay to the healthcare team to aid the decisions of discontinuing the medication, changing the route or dose of the antimicrobial, and planning for discharge.

The nurse contributes to discharge planning by providing patient and family education. Explicit instructions on monitoring for side effects and taking the medication as prescribed are essential components. The patient is advised to report any adverse reactions to the healthcare provider and continue with the antimicrobial for the full course. The duration of therapy is a balance between a course of treatment that is most effective for the shortest length of time and prevention of a reinfection that may be resistant to further treatments. Taking antimicrobials with food is often included in the education to prevent gastrointestinal discomfort. Probiotics, supplements, or food containing microorganisms can help promote diversity of beneficial bacteria, prevent antimicrobial resistance, and minimize antimicrobial-associated diarrhea.

The nurse also plays an important role in surgical antimicrobial stewardship, which includes measures to prevent additional antimicrobial therapy due to surgical site infections (SSI). Preoperatively, the patient is instructed and/or assisted to cleanse the body with an antimicrobial soap. The nurse advocates for the optimal antimicrobial prophylaxis selection for the procedure, dose, frequency, and timing. Medication administration is communicated with the perioperative nurse. During surgery, infection control measures include hand hygiene, appropriate PPE, surgical site preparation with an antiseptic agent, glycemic control, oxygen administration, prevention of hypothermia, and proper cleaning and sterilization of equipment. Postoperatively, the nurse provides wound care using aseptic technique, encourages good nutrition to aid in wound healing, administers oxygen as ordered, and monitors the patient's temperature and general health condition.

Medication Management

Safe Medication Administration Practices

Rights of Drug Administration

Ensuring medication safety is a fundamental nursing responsibility. Although pharmacological interventions are considered therapeutic, can alleviate suffering, and also aid in healing, the potential for harm still exists. The nurse uses clinical judgment, applies nursing and pharmacological knowledge, and makes decisions with every medication administration. Traditionally, the five medication rights provide a basic foundation to guide patient safety. These rights include the right patient, right drug, right dose, right route, and right time/frequency.

The right patient prompts the nurse to consider whether the correct person is being given the medication. Two patient identifiers (e.g., name and date of birth) are used with every medication pass. With the right drug, the nurse verifies that the correct medication is ordered by the healthcare provider and administered to the patient. The right dose confirms that the amount given is appropriate for the patient, with consideration to age, weight, and provider order parameters. The nurse also notes that the medication route is appropriate for the patient, including the site of administration. If the drug route is oral, the nurse would consider any swallowing difficulties or an NPO status that requires a different

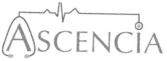

route. Finally, the nurse makes sure to administer the drug at the right time, which is within a specified time range per institutional policy and may apply to meal times.

The medication rights that guide practice are extended to include the right reason, right documentation, and right response. The nurse verifies the right reason, medication purpose, and correct circumstance in which the medication is administered. With the right documentation, the nurse documents administration upon providing the medication. Finally, the nurse evaluates the right response, including any efficacious medication outcome or side effect.

Barcode medication administration (BMA) contributes to patient safety, although it is not a substitution for the five rights. BMA is a system in which the nurse scans the patient identification wristband and the medication barcode as part of the electronic record. The computer identifies the patient, medication, dose, and time administered. Barcoding can decrease the amount of human error. However, clinical judgment is needed in order to consider the entire landscape of medication administration to prevent harm.

The process of medication administration does not end with the intervention of providing the patient with the pharmacological treatment. After the medication is documented, the outcome is evaluated. Side effects and allergic reactions may occur in time and likely warrant further follow-up.

Steps for Safe Medication Administration

The steps of medication administration are imperative to provide patient safety beyond the five medication rights. Although the five rights framework serves as a foundation for safety, the patient may still be susceptible to medication error. With consideration given to the patient's clinical condition, work environment, and other distractions, the nurse is constantly using critical thinking and clinical judgment to ensure safe medication administration.

Errors can occur from the initiation of a medication order. The nurse first reviews the provider order to verify that the medication is reasonable for the particular patient, with the correct dose and frequency. Patient allergies are both verified with the patient and reviewed in the medical record before medications are given. The nature of the allergic response, such as a hypersensitivity response or a non-life-threatening side effect, is important to consider. The nurse communicates with the provider and/or the pharmacist about any questions needing answers or clarification required.

When preparing medications, the environment should be quiet, with minimal distractions. One patient's medication is prepared at a time. The medication is scrutinized to ensure that the packaging is intact, the medication is not expired, and the medication name is correct. Look-alike/sound-alike errors can occur when names look or sound similar. If administering an intravenous medication, the amount and type of diluent used for reconstitution should be accurate.

The individual patient and their clinical condition are also considered. Focused assessments are often necessary, according to the situation. For example, a cardiovascular assessment that includes vital signs is completed prior to administering cardiac medications. Cardiac medications may not be warranted if the heart rate and/or blood pressure is too low. A pain assessment would be performed prior to pain medication administration. Lab values may be affected by the drug, in particular electrolytes and renal function. If furosemide is ordered and the serum potassium is low, replacement potassium is often required. Written parameters may be available with the order for the nurse to follow. The nurse communicates with the physician if there are any concerns about the focused assessment. Once the patient is given the medication, they are assessed during and after administration for any adverse effects, especially if the treatment is new.

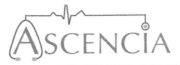

Drug Interactions

In many cases, medical-surgical patients take a variety of different medications, including new pharmacological treatments. The nurse plays a pivotal role in recognizing drug-drug and food-drug interactions to prevent any adverse reactions. Often, computer systems provide alerts and warnings prior to administration of a drug with a potential interaction. However, these notifications may also lead to alert fatigue when there is an abundance of warnings. Despite automated warnings, the nurse remains vigilant in referencing drug reference guides to review any potential interactions. With intravenous medications, the nurse confirms that piggyback medication may be administered with a continuous fluid order.

Polypharmacy can lead to the possibility of medication harm with respect to drug-drug interactions. One drug may work a certain way in the body. However, if another drug is administered, there may be potential for an unsuspected side effect that would not occur if the drugs were given separately. Another medication may be added to address the new side effect, leading to a prescribing cascade and potential for more interactions and synergism. Furthermore, a drug interaction may affect the absorption, metabolism, elimination, or bioavailability of a drug. For example, one drug may not work as well or may reach toxic levels. Additionally, especially in the elderly population, drug interactions may lead to cognitive changes, increased falls, readmissions, and overall increased morbidity and mortality.

Certain foods can interact with medications in a similar manner, affecting the pharmacokinetic or pharmacodynamic properties of the drug. One example is that of warfarin. When patients consume a high amount of vitamin K, found in green leafy vegetables, the intended effect of warfarin is lessened. If patients are administered a monoamine oxidase inhibitor (MAOI), foods high in tyramine (e.g., cheese) can lead to a hypertensive crisis. Sometimes, a patient is advised to take medication on an empty stomach because the drug absorption may be affected, as with levothyroxine. Other times, food is advised to prevent gastric irritation. The nurse has an important responsibility to provide education to the patient regarding food-drug interactions. The patient must be aware of how to care for themselves at home and communicate any dietary needs to others.

Adverse Reactions

When taking any medication, the patient may experience an unwanted symptom as a result. This symptom, whether mild or serious, may impact the patient's quality of life and require additional intervention. A side effect is considered an unplanned yet commonly known result of taking a drug, regardless of dosage. It is not an intended consequence. For instance, a side effect of lisinopril is a lingering cough. An adverse drug reaction (ADR) is an undesired and/or harmful outcome of the pharmacological drug despite taking the medication as prescribed. An ADR results in some form of injury. As a result, the patient seeks medical care, causing emergency room visits, hospitalization, longer hospital stays, and/or death. For example, a patient taking an anticoagulant may experience a hemorrhage, which may be life-threatening.

The nurse plays a pivotal role in recognizing any adverse reactions. The bedside nurse has the ability to recognize unintended effects promptly because of the amount of time spent with the patient. Once the nurse administers the medication, the outcome is monitored and documented. Part of the professional responsibility of the nurse is to be knowledgeable about medications, the medications' side effects and potential adverse reactions, and any changes in the patient's clinical condition. Nurses are constantly monitoring patients' cognition, vital signs, and reports of problems. When a patient's clinical condition deteriorates, which may be seen with anaphylaxis, somnolence, or acute bleeding episodes, the nurse responds by activating the Rapid Response Team and/or notifying the provider. Furthermore, the nurse

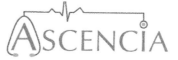

has the duty to educate the patient about their medications. When patients are discharged, they must know about the signs of adverse reactions and the necessary follow-up (e.g., notifying the physician, calling 911, returning to the hospital).

Other related terms are adverse events and sentinel events. Adverse drug events (ADEs) encompass adverse drug reactions as well as other unplanned harm, which is often temporary. These may include drug overdoses, injury due to discontinuation (i.e., withdrawal), and medication error. On the other hand, a sentinel event causes permanent harm, damage, and/or injury, including death that is not the result of the disease process itself.

Patient Medication Education

Nurses provide education on prescribed medications to improve patient autonomy, the patient's decision-making ability, and overall health outcomes. When patients do not receive sufficient education, they may not understand the medication instructions or recognize important side or adverse effects; they may even delay seeking treatment. As a result, patients are at risk for mishandling medication, readmission, or complications. Patient teaching begins once the medication is ordered and continues upon administration and through discharge.

When teaching is planned, the patient's preferred learning style is identified. For example, patients who like to read may value handouts, those who are visual learners may request a video, and auditory learners may choose to listen. Some medications, such as insulin or injectable anticoagulants, are taught in a hands-on manner. During education, teach-back is used. The patient is prompted to describe the information according to their own understanding. The nurse uses objective questions to have the patient describe what they were taught.

Patient comprehension of instructions facilitates the proper use of medication. Understanding prescriptions helps prevent patient harm and provides guidelines for follow-up with the medical provider. It is important to consider the patient's health literacy and cognitive function. Educational material should be written at a level comprehensible to the patient. If the patient's cognitive function is not conducive to teaching, the family or caregiver should be involved whenever possible. For example, the daughter of a geriatric patient with dementia could receive teaching. Even if the patient does not have any cognitive impairments, they may request that a family member or other caregiver also receive education for extra support.

Technology is an integral aspect of personalized patient education. The nurse uses organizational software to print health literature, which may be customized for a particular language. Apps can provide instruction about the clinical condition or medication. Tablets, in-room televisions, and other devices can play videos that explain complex medical processes. These tools aid in achieving positive patient outcomes. Additionally, nurses use technology to document education to build upon the continuity of teaching.

Polypharmacy

Medication Reconciliation

Medication reconciliation is the method of collecting a complete and accurate list of a patient's medications. The list contains full drug information (name, dose, frequency, and route) and encompasses prescribed medications, over-the-counter drugs, supplements, and vitamins. During this process, medications are verified, reviewed for drug interactions and therapeutic value, and considered for discontinuation. As a key opportunity to prevent adverse drug events, medication reconciliation

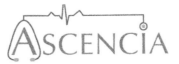

ensures that drugs are not omitted or duplicated and validates that medication lists are current and accurate. Furthermore, drugs may be discontinued by the provider if the medication is no longer necessary.

A standardized process for medication reconciliation within the healthcare system decreases adverse drug events. For example, one department has the main responsibility of collecting medication reconciliation data. Documentation is timely and readily accessible in the medical record for nurses, pharmacists, and healthcare providers to review. The list provides the opportunity to compare the healthcare provider's medication orders at any transition time (i.e., admission, transfer, discharge). Transitions of care represent vulnerable opportunities for medication error. For example, a patient is admitted to the hospital with a history of hypertension, yet the cardiac medication he typically takes at home is not ordered. Because of this omission, the patient may experience a cerebrovascular accident.

Medication reconciliation is vital because medication harm is a culprit of readmissions, morbidity, and mortality. Obtaining a complete and accurate medication reconciliation list is important for every healthcare visit. One consequence of an incomplete medication reconciliation is the inability to identify polypharmacy. Polypharmacy is defined as taking at least five medications in the home environment and over ten medications during hospitalization. The potential outcomes of multiple medications are adverse drug events, drug interactions, and medication errors. Common in older adults due to chronic conditions, polypharmacy can lead to falls, delirium, frailty, a lessened ability to live independently, increased hospitalization, decreased quality of life, and a higher risk of mortality. When an accurate list of medications is available, polypharmacy can be addressed to eliminate drugs not clinically indicated. For instance, medications that have a tendency to cause adverse events in the geriatric population are anticholinergics and narcotics. The healthcare team has the opportunity to review the benefits and negative consequences with the patient and consider alternative choices.

Interdisciplinary Communication

In the hospital environment, medication reconciliation takes place during admission, transfers to different levels of care, and discharge as well as throughout the shift. Often, the interprofessional team (the nurse, pharmacist, and healthcare provider) is involved in data collection by interviewing the patient, verifying current medication lists with the patient's pharmacy, and/or confirming medication with caregivers. According to institutional policy, one department may have the primary responsibility of completing this process.

Communication among the interdisciplinary team provides a comprehensive overview of prescribed medications. Discussions allow for consideration of the number of medications, benefits and drawbacks, clinical indication and proper dosage, alternative treatments, applicable monitoring (labs, vital signs), adverse drug reactions, and best options according to evidence-based practice. In order to effectively address polypharmacy, the healthcare provider discontinues medication that has more harm than benefit or has ambiguous outcomes. For drugs that may present withdrawal effects, the patient requires tapering of medications or follow-up monitoring.

Managing polypharmacy is an important coordinated responsibility of the interdisciplinary team. As the prescriber, the healthcare provider is in the position of overseeing the ordering and discontinuing of medications and optimizing the drugs prescribed. Pharmacists verify and dispense medications. They have the expertise to identify drug-drug interactions, adverse effects, and improper doses while also providing valuable education to patients and interdisciplinary team members. The nurse plays a pivotal role in coordinating medication reconciliation. In addition to reviewing the medication list, discrepancies are clarified with the healthcare provider. Because of constant communication with the patient, the

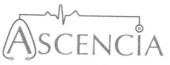

nurse may be the recipient of medication concerns or questions that can be relayed to the healthcare team. They also establish educational goals and provide routine teaching to the patient.

Safe Drug Management and Disposal

Medication Storage

The storage of medication within a healthcare facility serves to protect not only the drug but also the patient. Specific processes may vary by state regulations and institutional policies. Environmental factors, including temperature, moisture, and light exposure, can degrade drugs. The drugs are kept in a climate-controlled area within a certain temperature range recommended by the manufacturer so that their efficacy is maintained. Some medications require refrigeration. For example, opened bottles of Humulin R cannot be exposed to heat or light, and unopened bottles require refrigeration.

Storage also requires a secured space to prevent tampering, mishandling, or contamination and to maintain an accurate count for supply. Medications must be safeguarded from unauthorized personnel and the generalized patient population. Many institutions utilize an automated dispensing cabinet. The cabinet and individual drawers are locked until the nurse withdraws the medication. In addition to the medication count, it is also critical that any drug withdrawal, waste, and returns be tracked. Before administering medications to patients, the drugs are kept in their original packaging and clearly labeled.

Controlled substances require additional stipulations to prevent tampering and diversion. Narcotics are maintained in supervised areas with medication room doors closed and locked. These drugs have their own locked storage container within the automated dispensing cabinet and refrigerator. The nurse is prompted to count the number of medications in the container prior to removing the drug. When administering the medication, the nurse directly observes the patient taking it. If the patient is not ready to take the drug, the medication is stored and locked.

In the home environment, storage of prescription drugs is an important aspect of discharge teaching. Medications are kept within a specific temperature range according to the manufacturer. Typically, drugs are stored at 59–86°F or 15–30°C, with a relative humidity below 60 percent. Certain locations may affect the drug's integrity. For example, bathrooms tend to have high humidity. The room chosen should have a suitable, consistently maintained climate-controlled environment.

Securing home medications is a safety priority. Medication should be stored out of reach and not visible to those at high risk for harming themselves, especially children and people with cognitive impairments. When medications are easily accessible, there is a higher risk of harm among these populations, including accidental overdose or poisoning. Additionally, unused medications can easily accumulate, which creates the potential for sharing prescriptions with household members for whom the drug was not prescribed. Medications should be stored separately from the medications of others in the household, in a secure location, and in the original container with the affixed label; expired medications should be disposed of.

Medication Disposal

Pharmaceutical waste is a safety concern in the healthcare setting because of the risks of exposure to harmful chemicals, environmental pollution, and drug diversion. Disposal processes are often set in place according to regulatory guidelines, although they may vary by institutional policy. Proper disposal aims to prevent contamination of the water supply. Medication is classified according to nonhazardous, hazardous, and controlled substance waste and discarded in designated labeled bins. Nonhazardous medication includes over-the-counter drugs and chemicals determined to be nontoxic.

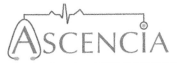

Hazardous pharmaceutical waste that includes specified agents (e.g., nitroglycerin tablets, nicotine patches, oxybutynin) is placed in a designated RCRA black bin. These items are in compliance with the Resource Conservation and Recovery Act—a regulation providing a management structure for pharmaceutical waste—, which is overseen by the Environmental Protection Agency (EPA).

Controlled substance waste is also regulated by federal agencies, including the Drug Enforcement Administration (DEA). Regulations state that the drug cannot be flushed, must be destroyed, and must not be retrievable. A separate designated container can destroy and denature the pharmaceutical drug through a chemical process. These drugs also require a second nurse witness when wasting.

The nurse educates the patient about the proper disposal of medications when at home. Patients are directed to read the instructions on the prescription drug label, package insert, or medication teaching sheet. Flushing of medications down the toilet or sink is frequently not advised. The U.S. Drug and Food Administration (FDA) recommends that drug take-back programs be utilized. These programs include a wide variety of options, such as bringing the drugs to community collection receptacles or community drug take-back events, conferring with the local pharmacy, or participating in mail-back programs.

However, if the patient is not able to access a designated site, then flushing the substance down the toilet may be advisable if the drug is listed on the FDA flush list. Because drugs may be toxic or fatal to others, flushing would be the safest method in some instances. If the drug is not on the flush list, the patient should follow recommended guidelines per the FDA regulations. These include mixing the drug with a dirt-like substance (e.g., cat litter, coffee grounds), enclosing the material in a sealed plastic bag, and disposing of the container in the household trash.

Advanced Access Devices

Peripheral Venous Catheter (PVC)

The majority of hospitalized patients receive short-term intravenous (IV) therapy during their admission. The IV route has many benefits, such as hydration through fluids, restoring electrolyte balance, delivering blood products, and administering medication. Unlike the oral route, in which drugs are gradually absorbed, IV medication is immediately bioavailable because of direct access to the systemic circulation. When patients cannot take medication orally, administering drugs intravenously provides an alternative option. IV administrations occur through intermittent or continuous infusions or through a bolus injection (IV push).

The knowledge and skill set of intravenous therapy (e.g., peripheral IV insertion, IV therapy administration) are imperative to safe patient care. When preparing for IV insertion, nursing activities include communicating with the patient, selecting the appropriate size catheter, positioning the patient, using aseptic technique, and choosing the ideal location. The nurse may have challenges inserting a peripheral IV due to a variety of patient factors, including age, cognitive factors (e.g., restlessness), skin pigmentation, obesity, previous IV drug use, hypotension, and limb restrictions.

After insertion, the nurse assesses the IV site for patency and observes for complications (e.g., infiltration, phlebitis). Proper preparation and administration of IV medications help reduce adverse events. The nurse is vigilant about infection control by preparing medication in a clean environment and maintaining the sterility of the product. Injectable medications are labeled clearly with patient and drug information when prepared away from the patient bedside. The proper diluent is used. The medication is administered using a rate according to manufacturer guidelines. When caring for the IV site, the dressing is changed when soiled or loose. The IV site is removed and rotated when clinically indicated or per institutional policy.

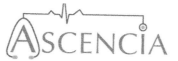

Common complications at the peripheral IV site are infection, infiltration, extravasation, and phlebitis. When an infection arises, erythema, warmth, and purulent drainage are often seen at the insertion site and along the vein. Infiltration occurs when the IV fluid or medication does not remain in the vein and leaks out into the surrounding tissue. Patients may report tenderness or pain. Swelling, coolness, and blanching are often noted. With extravasation, the fluid or medication that leaks out is a vesicant, causing tissue damage. When phlebitis takes place, the wall of the vein becomes inflamed. The vein may feel cordlike, with erythema and edema at the catheter site and along the vein.

Due to immediate drug bioavailability, complications with IV therapy administration can be serious. Medications given by IV bolus pose their own risk because they are more concentrated and administered rapidly. Adverse drug events can occur due to inaccurate drug calculations, inexperience with supplies and equipment, improper preparation and administration, and contamination.

Central Venous Catheter (CVC)

A central venous catheter (CVC) allows IV therapy infusion through a central vein (internal jugular, subclavian, or femoral vein) directly into the superior vena cava or cavoatrial junction. Clinical indications include the inability to obtain peripheral IV access, emergency situations, or when the situation warrants it (e.g., total parenteral nutrition, therapy irritating to peripheral veins, procedures such as continuous renal replacement therapy). The large central vein accessed allows for rapid infusions of therapies, obtaining blood samples, and hemodynamic monitoring. Upon insertion, the tip of the line is confirmed by X-ray prior to use. Multiple lumens allow for administering different intravenous therapies. If a CVC line is power injectable, contrast agents for radiology procedures can be injected through it. CVC lines are short-term, from a few days to several weeks.

CVC complications can vary, depending upon the site and the ability to perform ultrasound-guided placement. The most frequent are central line-associated bloodstream infections (CLABSI), thrombi, and emboli. The large veins are in close proximity to large arteries, and puncturing an artery can result in hemorrhage or emboli. The subclavian vein has a higher rate of pneumothorax due to its position near the clavicle and first rib. Although the femoral site may be the most accessible and away from other devices, it has high potential for CLABSI and is prone to thrombus formation.

Although the nurse does not insert a CVC, caring for the CVC is a nursing duty. The nurse performs an insertion site assessment, examining for erythema, edema, drainage, and dressing integrity. The dressing should be intact, clean, dry, and properly labeled (i.e., the date and time the dressing is placed). The line is assessed for patency by aspirating the catheter for blood return and determining any resistance. Dressing and needleless connector changes are completed per institutional policy. The dressing is changed using judicious infection control measures. The nurse performs hand hygiene, wears sterile gloves, and dons a mask and gown. Once the dressing is removed, the site is cleansed with chlorhexidine and allowed to dry. An antimicrobial transparent dressing is placed, the dressing is labeled, and a securement device is applied. CVC catheters are typically maintained and flushed according to institutional protocols, with low-dose heparin or normal saline used as a locking solution. Patient education is also essential, including infection prevention measures and safe handling.

Peripherally Inserted Central Venous Catheter (PICC)

A peripherally inserted central venous catheter (PICC) is a CVC that is inserted into a peripheral vein and terminates in the SVC or right atrium. Frequently, the PICC is placed in the basilic vein of the upper arm, although other veins can be used, including the brachial or cephalic veins. There are several benefits of using a PICC over another CVC line. PICCs can be used in both inpatient and outpatient settings for

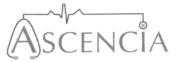

longer-term therapies up to several months. Complications are reduced because of insertion away from large arteries, and fewer infections are experienced. Common indications include administration of IV medications, blood products, therapies that cause irritation to peripheral veins, hyperosmolar solutions, and frequent lab draws.

The biggest complications of the PICC line are CLABSI, venous thromboembolism (VTE), and mechanical failure. Many procedures are in place to reduce the incidence of complications. These include utilizing an insertion checklist, employing maximum barrier precautions upon insertion, selecting catheters that minimize microbial colonization (e.g., polyurethane), choosing the lowest number of lumens required, cleansing the skin with a chlorhexidine preparation, using a chlorhexidine-impregnated transparent dressing, confirming the catheter tip location, referencing institutional flushing protocols and dressing change guidelines, and applying port protectors and securement devices.

A PICC line is often inserted by a specially trained nurse using ultrasound guidance. The tip of the PICC must be confirmed by X-ray or by an electrocardiogram-guided PICC placement. Confirmation by the latter method eliminates radiation and verifies placement using the maximum P amplitude on the electrocardiogram (ECG). Once the PICC is placed, the patient's limb use is restricted, and the nurse avoids taking blood pressures on that arm. Maintenance care is equivalent to the CVC line discussed above. The nurse assesses the insertion site for the appearance of erythema, edema, drainage, and dressing integrity. The PICC line lumens are flushed to ensure patency. When not in use, the line is locked with low-dose heparin or saline solution. Dressing changes and flushing frequency are determined by institutional policies. When occlusions are noted, fibrinolytic agents, such as alteplase, can be used. Patient education is imperative to ensure awareness of measures to minimize complications. These include infection prevention measures, signs/symptoms of complications, and handling the line with care.

Implanted Ports

Implanted ports are indicated when the patient requires an intermittent long-term infusion for months or years. Medical therapies that could warrant the use of an implanted port include chemotherapy, antibiotics, blood products, and/or intravenous fluids. During a surgical procedure, a catheter is inserted into a vein and secured by placement of a small port chamber in a subcutaneous pocket at the other end. The port is sealed under the skin by a silicone rubber septum.

Complications with implanted ports include infections, skin irritation, vein thrombosis, venous air embolism, and extravasation. Infections occur at the incision site or within the subcutaneous pocket. The patient may experience erythema, edema, warmth, fever, and purulent drainage. When a vein thrombosis occurs, swelling is present on the insertion side of the upper body (neck, face, shoulder, or arm), and there is a lack of blood return. A venous air embolism can lead to pulmonary and cardiovascular symptoms and increase mortality rates. Procedure-related complications include malposition, pneumothorax, thrombosis, and vein perforation. If extravasation occurs, the needle is likely dislodged into the subcutaneous tissue, causing discomfort and edema.

Accessing the port is completed in a series of steps. The nurse first performs hand hygiene and then dons a mask and sterile gloves. A non-coring needle is attached to a flushed extension set with a needleless connector. The access site is cleaned with a chlorhexidine scrub and allowed to dry. The nurse palpates the port with the nondominant gloved hand and stabilizes the port body. Then, the non-coring needle is inserted into the port body perpendicular to the back of the reservoir. Finally, the port is flushed with saline and aspirated for blood return. Once the needle is secured with sterile tape, a sterile transparent dressing is placed over the access site. The port is deaccessed once the locking solution has

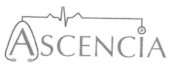

been administered. The nurse performs hand hygiene and dons gloves. The port septum is stabilized with the fingers of the nondominant hand, grasping either side of the port and pressing down. With the dominant hand, the non-coring needle is gripped and removed. The procedure is documented in the medical record.

The nurse cares for the implanted port site by assessing the insertion site for signs of infection. The line is flushed and locked with a locking solution during intermittent use. The dressing is changed when soiled or loose and according to institutional policies. Once the port is deaccessed, it is typically accessed once per month to be flushed and locked.

Epidurals

Often initiated in the surgical setting, an epidural provides the ability for anesthetics (e.g., bupivacaine) and analgesics (e.g., morphine, fentanyl) to be administered through the epidural space. A needle is inserted between two vertebrae into the region between the vertebral canal and the dura mater. The insertion may be in the cervical, thoracic, or lumbar spine, depending on the desired location for analgesia and/or anesthetic. The location is chosen according to the dermatomes that the sensory nerve roots innervate.

In the medical-surgical setting, the nurse cares for the patient receiving postoperative, post-procedural, or chronic pain management through an epidural. Drugs can be administered as a one-time bolus, as a continuous infusion, or via a patient-controlled epidural analgesia (PCEA) pump. In addition to pain control, other postoperative benefits include earlier ambulation, reduced risk of a cardiac event, decreased respiratory complications, improved bowel function, and shorter hospital lengths of stay.

Epidural complications arise due to catheter insertion problems or adverse reactions to the drugs administered. The insertion site can become infected. An epidural abscess or hematoma can occur. If the catheter migrates, the epidural may affect one side of the body. Patients can experience a postdural puncture headache, which happens if the needle punctures the dura mater. Furthermore, sensory and motor deficits can transpire as a result of the dermatomes innervated. If a patient has a reaction to the medication, symptoms can vary in severity. Examples include pruritus, nausea, vomiting, bradycardia, hypotension, urinary retention, and decreased level of consciousness. Opioid toxicity can ensue, which may lead to circumoral numbness, tinnitus, tremors, cardiac dysrhythmias, or seizures.

The nurse provides maintenance care for the epidural through careful nursing assessment, performed frequently at specified time intervals per institutional policy. Nursing responsibilities include monitoring vital signs, assessing pain levels, assessing insertion site appearance, assessing for nausea/vomiting, assessing for headache, assessing for urinary retention, monitoring the level of sedation, and monitoring for signs of toxicity. Motor and sensory assessments are performed to determine epidural effectiveness and identify complications. The epidural line is labeled, tubing is inspected for obstructions (i.e., kinks), and the line is traced prior to the patient receiving interventions. Dressings must be changed using strict aseptic technique, with any complications reported to the healthcare provider.

Financial Implications to Patients

Drug Assistance Programs

Pharmaceutical assistance programs (PAPs) can help low-income individuals who are uninsured or underinsured pay for prescription drugs. Along with government programs, pharmaceutical manufacturers and other nonprofit organizations may assist. Often, the type of insurance and medication are factors. Patients who are enrolled in Medicare may receive federal assistance with drug

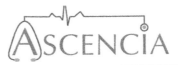

prescriptions. Drug plans can be added for patients who have Medicare Part A and/or Medicare Part B, which represent hospital and medical insurance. Other Medicare plans, such as Medicare Advantage Plan (Part C), offer drug coverage.

Available in some states, state PAPs (SPAPs) offer financial support for prescription drugs after other agencies are billed, such as Medicare, Medicaid, other private insurance, and/or federal programs. These programs vary by state. Apart from SPAPs, several states offer a discount program, in which the patient can pay a reduced cost.

Pharmaceutical manufacturers may sponsor PAPs to reduce patients' financial burden. Some have created their own private foundations and provide drugs to patients enrolled in certain private insurance or public health programs, such as Medicare Part D. Nonprofit organizations may provide prescription medication directly or offer financial assistance with qualified needs, such as the inability of the patient to pay the premium for their healthcare plan or meet copayments.

Interdisciplinary Communication

Interdisciplinary communication among the physician, nurse, pharmacist, case manager, and others can serve to strategize the patient costs of drug prescriptions in an effort to remove financial obstacles. The healthcare team communicates with the patient to ascertain whether prescriptions may be cost prohibitive. If patients do not share financial concerns, they may not fill the prescription or may skip doses of the medication. This can lead to ineffective management of the patient's health condition.

The team plans and coordinates discharge by reviewing the medication prescriptions required. One goal is to determine the medical necessity of the drug. If the medication is not advised, then deprescribing occurs by discontinuing or tapering the drug. Case managers are in a pivotal role of communicating with insurance companies and alerting the healthcare team if certain prescription drugs are not covered. A less costly alternative may be prescribed, which may involve avoiding brand name drugs. Some pharmacies offer certain generic medications at a low-cost value. Comparing pharmacies may result in finding prescription drugs at different costs.

Pain Management

Chronic and Acute Pain Management

Pain Assessment

When considering a pain assessment, the nurse understands that pain is a complex experience distinct to the individual. Many factors contribute to the experience of pain, including physical, social, and emotional factors. Considering that pain can directly affect the plan of care, the nurse plans goals for pain improvement, which often depend upon the situational context. For example, a goal planned for patients with chronic pain may be that the pain experienced is tolerable when engaging in activities.

A thorough assessment allows the nurse to determine the patient's level of comfort according to both subjective (e.g., patient report) and objective (e.g., respiratory rate, agitation) measures. Tools like the PQRST assessment tool prompt the nurse to ask detailed questions of responsive patients. The nurse engages in dialogue with the patient about the pain location, any causative factors, pain relief experienced, pain description (e.g., aching, burning, stabbing, dull, sharp, radiating), and timing (e.g.,

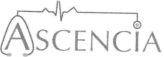

chronic, acute, constant, intermittent). Furthermore, the nurse ascertains how the patient is affected by the pain and whether routine activities, including mobility, are impacted.

Various pain severity rating scales are available. The scale selected should be appropriate for the patient's age and cognition, understandable to the nurse and patient, and a reasonable measurement of the experienced pain. The nurse considers the age of the patient, language barriers, and cognitive disturbances. For adult patients who are oriented, a common pain intensity scale is the Numerical Rating Scale (NRS), in which the patient is asked to rate their pain on a scale from 0 to 10 (with 0 being no pain and 10 being the worst pain). Patients who have difficulty providing a number may be asked to point to a visual face on a faces scale (e.g., Wong-Baker Faces scale) or use a visual analog to demonstrate pain severity. Visual scales are more appropriate than the NRS for children over the age of 3.

Although some pain rating scales provide important subjective information, their use alone may not capture the entire pain experience and may not be appropriate for some patients. For example, the NRS does not provide information about the patient's functional ability. Objective elements are addressed by certain situation-specific scales, including the Functional Pain Scale; the Face, Legs, Activity, Cry, Consolability (FLACC) scale for patients under 3; the Pain Assessment in Advanced Dementia (PAINAD) scale for adults with advanced dementia; and the Behavioral Pain Scale or Critical Care Pain Observation Tool (CPOT) for patients requiring ventilation. For instance, the PAINAD scale quantifies pain through assessment of breathing character (e.g., hyperventilation), negative vocalization (e.g., moaning), facial expression, body language, and consolability when a patient cannot communicate feelings of pain due to advanced dementia.

Pharmacological Treatment

Pharmacological treatment is considered once pain is thoroughly assessed and the treatment goals have been determined. The analgesic ladder, originally outlined by the World Health Organization (WHO) to address cancer pain, offers a pathway to reducing pain. The first step treats mild pain with nonopioid analgesics (e.g., nonsteroidal anti-inflammatory drugs [NSAIDs], acetaminophen). The second step uses weak opioids (e.g., codeine, hydrocodone), with nonopioid analgesics as needed, in the treatment of mild pain. Next, strong opioids (morphine, hydromorphone) are administered for severe and persistent pain, with additional nonopioid analgesics when needed. A non-pharmacological fourth step incorporates invasive and minimally invasive treatments (e.g., epidural analgesia, nerve blocks, palliation radiotherapy, spinal cord stimulation).

For each of these steps, adjuvants may be administered. Adjuvants used in pain management are drugs that may offer analgesic effects or enhance treatment when used with pain-relieving medications. The goal with adjuvants is to expand pharmacological approaches for individualized care. Examples include antidepressants (e.g., amitriptyline, nortriptyline) and anticonvulsants (e.g., gabapentin, carbamazepine). An adjuvant also provides an option if the intended medication did not provide relief.

With the concept of the analgesic ladder, the nurse assesses the patient's pain and administers the ordered medication at the lowest step possible. If pain reduction is not achieved, an adjuvant could be considered or a stronger medication from the next step could be provided. The analgesia is often started at the lowest dose, with a goal for the medication to last as long as possible. Patients may experience side effects and adverse reactions to the drugs, including opioid addiction. For example, NSAIDs may cause gastrointestinal disturbance. Patients who are opioid naïve, not having much prior exposure to this drug class, may experience respiratory depression or become too sedated. Careful monitoring and titrating of the medication allow the nurse to confirm how the drug will affect the patient.

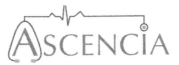

Documentation of pain medication administration, including pain assessment and reassessment, enhances communication within the medical record, supports decision-making, and provides continuity of care. With timely documentation, the nurse monitors the drug response, effectiveness, and adverse reactions. For some medications, close monitoring may be indicated. For example, because opioids can cause respiratory depression, the nurse monitors the patient's respiratory rate and uses clinical judgment to intervene as needed.

Non-Pharmacological Treatment

Non-pharmacological pain therapies offer a variety of options to aid in pain relief with minimal safety concerns. These are commonly referred to as complementary and alternative medicine (CAM) therapies. Benefits of CAM include holistic and personalized care, limited issues with side effects, and nominal financial expense. Often, these treatments aim to decrease stress and anxiety, improve mood, and encourage relaxation. As a result, patients often experience pain reduction and may require fewer pharmacological interventions.

In the hospital setting, the bedside nurse has the ability to implement CAM measures. Among the most common are repositioning and the use of ice and heat. Another nursing activity is assisting patients with ambulation. Increasing physical activity is correlated with decreased pain and improved functionality. Nursing units may offer comfort carts or comfort kits, which include items that can be tailored to patient preferences. Components can include aromatherapy through the use of essential oils, battery-operated candles, sleep masks, earplugs, MP3 players for guided imagery or music, and hand-held massage tools.

Various therapies may require further guidance from healthcare staff. Music therapy is often used in procedural settings and postoperatively for distraction and relaxation. Pet therapy, such as an animal-assisted therapy program, in which a dog provides visitation for short-term periods, may aid in pain management through improvement of the patient's mood and energy level. Reiki-trained nurses incorporate a modality in which their hands are placed near the patient's pain location with the use of energy to help decrease pain.

For chronic pain, therapies such as yoga, acupuncture, or biofeedback may be integrated. Yoga promotes the development of self-care skills and is considered an effective way to manage pain, anxiety, and depression. With acupuncture, an ancient form of healing, small needles are inserted into the skin to improve energy flow within the body. In biofeedback, devices measure physiological responses (e.g., heart rate, blood pressure, brainwaves) and provide timely feedback so that patients increase their awareness of these processes. Other therapies include diet changes, meditation, massage, and herbal medicine.

Patient Advocacy

When advocating for the patient suffering from pain, the nurse understands that pain may be profoundly subjective and deeply personal. The nurse has the ethical duty to decrease suffering, including the individual experience of pain. Pain management education is provided so that the patient is autonomous in their own treatment decisions. Information about intervention options, including pharmacological and non-pharmacological methods, medication dose and frequency ordered, side effects, and adverse reactions, is disclosed. The nurse supports beneficence by readily communicating with the patient and administering pain treatment in a timely manner. By intervening when the patient reports pain symptoms, the nurse applies the principle of nonmaleficence so that healing is not impeded. With respect to the ethical duty of justice, all patients are treated fairly and equally, regardless of any biases that may be present.

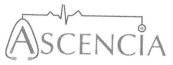

Despite the ethical duty of the nurse, pain interventions can also present complex situations. The nurse may be fearful of causing harm by intervening with pharmacological therapies, such as overmedicating a patient or contributing to addiction. Biases may be present because of previous personal or professional experiences. Moral disengagement, or the disassociation of ethical standards from a certain situation without feeling remorse, can occur. For example, the nurse may put ethical principles aside and not provide the patient with a certain pain intervention when he constantly rings the call light asking for more medication. Patients may be labeled as attention seeking or abusing narcotics with constant reports of pain, even with medication administration.

Because pain is multifaceted, a multimodal pain management strategy uses both pharmacological and non-pharmacological methods for treatment. With many different factors contributing to pain (e.g., the patient's medical history, perceptions of pain, root cause, or symptoms), a variety of options may be explored. This approach constitutes a holistic view of physical, psychological, and social components. In addition to the pain management methodologies already discussed, other examples include cognitive behavioral therapy to teach coping strategies, pain management education, and physical therapy. The goal is to adequately balance the management of pain, enhance the patient's quality of life, and produce a positive patient experience.

Surgical/Procedural Nursing Management

Pre-Procedural and Post-Procedural Standards

Pre-Procedural Universal Protocol

The purpose of the universal protocol is to prevent patient harm during surgical procedures. Errors in surgery, such as wrong-site, wrong-procedure, and wrong-person errors, can lead to serious consequences. Furthermore, the patient is unable to participate in care after receiving anesthesia and/or sedating medications. The three main components of the universal protocol encompass pre-procedure verification, site marking, and timeout.

Pre-procedure verification confirms that the procedure, patient, and surgical site are all accurate. The patient is involved in this process when possible. The items required for surgery are confirmed to be available and matched to the patient. These include documentation (e.g., history and physical, signed consent form), diagnostic and imaging results (e.g., radiology images and reports, biopsy reports), and anticipated supplies during surgery (e.g., blood products, special devices or equipment). If the patient is admitted to the inpatient unit, the nurse initiates preparation through the use of a preoperative checklist. For example, the nurse verifies that the history and physical evidence is present, the latest laboratory work is available, and an electrocardiogram is completed as indicated.

Site marking refers to marking the procedural site prior to surgery. If different locations are possible (e.g., an arm or leg), marking is essential to prevent the harm of a wrong-site surgery. An institutional process is followed, such as using a specific visible mark and confirming the site with the patient. Marking is completed by the accountable practitioner who will be present with the patient during surgery. For some sites that are not possible to mark (e.g., perineum, mucosal surfaces, teeth), institutional policies should be followed.

Before the procedure begins, a timeout occurs. During the timeout, the final patient identification and procedure verification are performed. Each facility establishes a standardized procedure. For example,

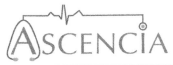

all timeouts are conducted with a designated leader and surgical team who will be present when the surgery begins. In a perioperative environment, this consists of a registered nurse circulator, surgical scrub nurse, surgeon, anesthesiologist, and any other applicable healthcare professional. The participants are focused on the timeout procedure without distractions. At the very least, the patient information, surgical site, and surgical procedure are jointly agreed upon. Other elements may include patient positioning, safety precautions, medication received, and equipment needed. All concerns must be settled prior to the surgery commencing. The timeout is documented as completed in the medical record. Although the timeout is used in the perioperative environment, it is frequently extended to other areas (e.g., interventional radiology, endoscopy, catheterization laboratory) where an invasive procedure is performed. Timeouts can also be performed at the bedside for procedures like central line placements.

Post-Procedural Monitoring

Once the procedure or surgery is completed, the patient is admitted into the post-anesthesia care unit (PACU) upon transfer of care. While patients recovering from general or regional anesthesia are admitted to the PACU, intubated or critically ill patients may be recovered in the intensive care unit (ICU). Close monitoring is required due to the effects of the procedure or the sedation or anesthesia received. This occurs in two stages of recovery, early (PACU phase 1) and late (PACU phase 2). During early recovery, anesthesia recovery and restoration of baseline vital signs are the goals. In late recovery, the PACU nurse focuses on transitioning the patient to the nursing unit or, if applicable, the home environment.

Patients are assessed and closely monitored to prevent complications (e.g., pneumonia, hemorrhage, hypothermia, hypovolemia or hypervolemia, infection). Specific criteria must be met prior to the PACU discharge according to institutional procedure. Patients must perform certain life-sustaining functions, such as breathing on their own and regaining sensation and motor activity. Vital signs are assessed every 15 minutes initially, with a goal of baseline restoration and appropriate thermoregulation. The patient's temperature should be maintained between 96.8°F/36°C and 100.4°F/38°C.

The nurse frequently conducts a comprehensive assessment to meet discharge criteria goals. Neurologically, the patient should be alert, awake, and arousable to stimuli, with baseline orientation. Assessment of circulation should show that the patient is hemodynamically stable, without signs of active bleeding or blood loss. With the respiratory assessment, the patient should be able to breathe spontaneously on their own, maintain a patent airway with appropriate functioning of reflexes (e.g., coughing, swallowing), and sustain blood oxygenation with SpO_2 greater than or equal to 92% on room air. Urine output should be sufficient—greater than 30 mL/hour.

Additionally, the PACU nurse ensures that pain is tolerable with adequate pain control measures and postoperative nausea and vomiting is controlled. Skin integrity at the procedural site is assessed and monitored for excessive drainage. In order to discharge the patient, facility-defined scoring systems (e.g., Aldrete) should be properly used.

Pertinent Potential Complications and Management

Respiratory Complications

General anesthesia leads to loss of physiological functions (e.g., consciousness, autonomic reflexes) that support adequate ventilation. To maintain a patent airway, an endotracheal (ET) tube is inserted intraoperatively, through which breaths can be delivered via mechanical ventilation. Consequently,

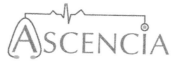

respiratory complications may develop. Contributing factors include preexisting health conditions (e.g., morbid obesity, obstructive sleep apnea [OSA], chronic obstructive pulmonary disease [COPD], dysphagia), preoperative medications (e.g., central nervous system depressants, gabapentin, pregabalin), intraoperative opioids, and prolonged length of surgery. When the patient transitions from anesthesia to the conscious state, these factors may affect the recovery of respiratory muscles and the respiratory drive.

Aspiration occurs when foreign contents (e.g., gastric contents) enter the lungs and produce respiratory complications. Inhalation of gastric contents causes aspiration pneumonitis, inflammation from chemical burns in the airway and lungs. Often due to a decreased level of consciousness from anesthesia, symptoms may include oxygen desaturation, pulmonary edema, cyanosis, shortness of breath, and acute respiratory distress. As a preventive measure, patients refrain from eating or drinking prior to surgery for a specified number of hours. Aspiration pneumonia is the infectious process caused by pathogenic bacteria when oropharyngeal secretions enter the lungs. Signs and symptoms are fever, tachypnea, and cough. Preoperative oral care measures can reduce infection risk. Postoperatively, dysphagia screening (i.e., a monitored sip test) identifies aspiration. Treatment may include suctioning, supplemental oxygen, antibiotics, nasogastric tube placement, and reintubation.

Laryngospasm is an emergent respiratory complication. Although this protective mechanism prevents pulmonary aspiration, a partial or complete closure of the glottis leads to airway obstruction. Gas exchange becomes impeded, which may result in pulmonary edema or death. Causes include secretions, foreign object stimulation (e.g., oral airway), or intraoperative vocal cord irritation. The goal is to remove the irritation and urgently open the airway through positive-pressure ventilation with a bag valve mask. The patient may be given a muscle paralytic drug (i.e., succinylcholine) to halt the laryngospasm. Reintubation and mechanical ventilation may be required, necessitating a higher level of care postoperatively and a longer length of stay (LOS). Once the airway is patent, the goal is to maintain the airway and deliver supplemental oxygen to ensure sufficient oxygenation.

Hypoventilation is caused by CO_2 retention. Consequently, the patient may experience hypoxemia and hypercapnia. The etiology may be related to the effects of anesthesia drugs (e.g., opioids, neuromuscular blocking agents) that depress the respiratory drive, ventilation muscle weakness, pain, and agitation. Signs are $PaCO_2 > 50$ mmHg or a respiratory rate of < 8 breaths/min. Maintaining a patent airway is a crucial goal. Patients are monitored by a pulse oximeter and treated with supplemental oxygen but may require noninvasive bilevel positive airway pressure (BiPAP) or reintubation and mechanical ventilation in severe cases.

Cardiovascular Complications

During surgery, hemodynamic status is influenced by several factors, such as anesthesia, fluid administration, and blood loss. Cardiac output is crucial for maintaining perfusion to vital organs and tissues. Any changes relating to this mechanism (e.g., blood volume, stroke volume, heart rate) consequently affect the patient's blood pressure and cardiac rhythm. Consider the patient receiving intraoperative intravenous fluid. The added volume increases cardiac output, which increases blood pressure. Whether blood vessels are dilated or constricted has bearing on perfusion. The cardiac conduction system allows the heart to pump properly. If the patient experiences a cardiac dysrhythmia, cardiac output decreases. Conversely, if the patient has decreased cardiac output, then a dysrhythmia (e.g., atrial fibrillation, supraventricular tachycardia) can occur.

Hypotension is characterized as a systolic blood pressure (SBP) of less than 90 mmHg and/or mean arterial pressure (MAP) of less than 60 mm Hg, or a decrease in the patient's baseline of these values of

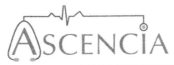

at least 10%. Among the causes are drug side effects (e.g., anesthesia, antibiotics, antihypertensives), hypovolemia due to volume depletion or bleeding, sepsis, tissue manipulation, clamping of blood vessels, and heart failure. The nurse monitors vital signs and pulse oximetry and identifies signs of inadequate tissue perfusion (e.g., cyanosis, low urine output). Treatment is aimed at reversing the cause and restoring hemodynamic stability. This may include fluid resuscitation, medication administration (e.g., ephedrine, epinephrine), holding antihypertensives, administering blood products, and reducing tissue retraction. Complications include myocardial injury, acute renal failure, and death.

Hypertension occurs from anxiety, preexisting chronic conditions (e.g., hypertension, renal disease), increased pain, urinary retention, fluid overload, and anesthetic drugs (e.g., ketamine). Often, patients are considered hypertensive with SBP > 170 mmHg or diastolic blood pressure (DPB) > 100. Prior to surgery, antihypertensives (e.g., beta-blockers, calcium channel blockers) may be administered. The surgical team monitors the patient's blood pressure and implements other perioperative interventions when necessary (e.g., pain medications, urinary catheter insertion for urinary retention). Hypertensive complications include heart failure, stroke, and acute renal failure.

The complication of cardiac dysrhythmias may increase with preexisting cardiac disease. There are a variety of causes, such as anesthetic agents, surgery location (e.g., cardiac surgery), vagal stimulation, electrolyte imbalances, intubation, pain, hypothermia, hypoxemia, and fluid overload. Dysrhythmias lead to increased risk of further complications, such as poor hemodynamic stability, blood clots, and stroke. Common dysrhythmias are atrioventricular (AV) block, atrial fibrillation, atrial flutter, paroxysmal supraventricular tachycardia, premature ventricular contraction, ventricular tachycardia, ventricular fibrillation, and torsade de pointes. The intervention depends upon the particular rhythm. For example, cardiac medications (e.g., amiodarone, beta-blockers) are administered with atrial fibrillation to control the heart rate, and cardioversion is performed if drugs are unsuccessful. If the patient experiences cardiac arrest, then cardiopulmonary resuscitation (CPR) is initiated.

Complications of the Central Nervous System

Perioperative complications of the central nervous system transpire as a result of anesthesia, sedating drugs, or disruption of normal physiological processes during surgery. Clearance of anesthesia can be delayed due to the patient's age or preexisting conditions (e.g., renal or hepatic disease) and prolonged intubation. Surgery may interfere with tissue oxygenation, nutrient delivery, and cellular waste removal. Severe neurological consequences include stroke, seizures, and brain injury. Two common negative outcomes are delirium and thermoregulation impairment.

Delirium is characterized by a temporary altered level of consciousness (LOC), common among the elderly. The condition occurs within 2 days after surgery. Patients may exhibit characteristics that are hypoactive (e.g., decreased LOC, slow speech, reduced movement) or hyperactive (e.g., inability to maintain attention, agitation, disorientation, perceptual disturbances, memory impairment, disorganized thinking). Preexisting conditions (e.g., age, nutritional deficiencies, cognitive impairments) or effects of hospitalization (e.g., medication, electrolyte imbalances, pain, immobility, interference in the sleep/wake cycle) are contributing factors. Because of the subtle signs and symptoms, nurses use a delirium screening tool like the Confusion Assessment Method (CAM) and a sedation scale, such as the Richmond Agitation-Sedation Scale (RAAS), to detect postoperative delirium. Interventions include providing the patient's eyeglasses and hearing aids, correcting electrolyte imbalances, holding medications that worsen delirium, providing sufficient pain control, implementing early mobility, and discontinuing indwelling urinary catheters early. Delirium contributes to a longer LOS and increased risk of aspiration, cognitive disorders, and mortality.

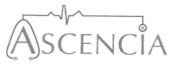

Hypothermia, defined as a temperature of less than 36°C /96.8°F, results from environmental or surgical factors (e.g., operating room temperature, administration of cool intravenous fluids, anesthetic drugs, loss of body heat, increased length of surgery). Even mild decreases in body temperature may lead to complications related to blood coagulation and blood loss. Vasoconstriction impedes tissue oxygenation, which can consequently impair wound healing and cause surgical site infections (SSIs). Nursing interventions include proactive monitoring of the patient's temperature, anticipating temperature loss by implementing warming measures (e.g., warming blanket), and providing oxygen to meet increased oxygenation demands.

Malignant hyperthermia (MH) is a life-threatening complication, with a classic sign of an elevated temperature, often progressing rapidly. Caused by a genetic trait that affects the response to anesthetic drug exposure, MH leads to a hypermetabolic state, extreme release of calcium by skeletal muscle cells, and muscle rigidity. Increased oxygen consumption and heat production result. Vital organs are compromised once the temperature approaches 41.5°C/106.7°F. Signs and symptoms include fever, hypertension, tachypnea, hypercapnia, hypoxia, hyperkalemia, metabolic acidosis, arrhythmias, and jaw muscle rigidity. Disseminated intravascular coagulation (DIC) and end-stage organ failure can ensue from rhabdomyolysis and acidosis. Interventions include the administration of a muscle relaxant (e.g., dantrolene), initiating cooling measures, and correcting acidosis, arrhythmias, and electrolyte imbalances.

Gastrointestinal Complications

The effects of surgery can potentiate gastrointestinal (GI) complications, including postoperative nausea and vomiting (PONV) and constipation. PONV risk factors are female sex, history of motion sickness, length and type of surgery, prolonged fasting time, medications (e.g., opioids), and anxiety. Often, prophylactic treatment is administered. Pharmacological interventions include antiemetics (e.g., ondansetron, scopolamine transdermal, promethazine, metoclopramide), alternative pain-relieving medication if opioids induce nausea, and intravenous fluids. The nurse also implements non-pharmacological nursing interventions like stimulation of the P6 acupressure point or aromatherapy. PONV results in delayed nutrition, dehydration, longer LOS, and patient dissatisfaction.

Constipation can be common in later stages of postoperative care due to the type of surgery, narcotic administration, lack of intake, and decreased mobility. Other risk factors include female sex, emotional factors, low fiber and fluid intake, and medical history. Indications of constipation are abdominal distention, nausea, and inability to eliminate stool. The nurse provides patient education and implements measures of early mobility, increasing fluid and fiber intake and avoiding bedpans, prudent use of pain medication, and administration of stool softeners and laxatives.

A common cause of both nausea and vomiting postoperatively, as well as constipation, is a paralytic ileus. This condition is the cessation of intestinal motility without mechanical obstruction. Signs are absent bowel sounds, lack of flatus, and abdominal distention. Because contents are not moving through the gut, patients experience increased pain, nausea and vomiting, constipation, and bloating. Interventions include early mobilization, early discontinuation of indwelling urinary catheters, and limited use of nasogastric tubes (NGTs). Motility often recovers within 3 days, but further complications are decreased nutritional intake and electrolyte imbalances.

Additional Postoperative Risks

In the postoperative period, patients may be at risk for additional complications, such as uncontrolled pain, infections, and falls. When pain management efforts are not successful, patients can experience

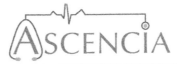

complications in every system. Patients are less apt to increase mobility, take deep breaths, and eat. Physiological symptoms like tachycardia, hypoventilation, ileus, nausea and vomiting, and/or urinary retention may occur. Severe complications include myocardial infarction, poor immune function, delayed wound healing, and decreased quality of life. Nurses can implement multimodal analgesia, combining opioid and nonopioid analgesics, adjuvants, and non-pharmacological measures.

Postoperative infections consist of surgical site infections, catheter-associated urinary tract infections (CAUTI), and pneumonia. General signs and symptoms of infection are fever, increased white blood cell count, and tachycardia. The wound appearance is monitored for increased tenderness, edema, and drainage character. Interventions include obtaining a wound culture, administering antibiotics, and performing wound care. To prevent CAUTI, early discontinuation of the indwelling urinary catheter decreases risk. The nurse assesses for urinary retention and assists with scheduled toileting. Signs of pneumonia include cough, tachypnea, shortness of breath, and excessive sputum production. The nurse encourages coughing, deep breathing, and the use of an incentive spirometer. Early mobility and oral hygiene are important measures in pneumonia prevention.

Patients are at risk for falling due to a variety of factors. The experience of incisional pain and discomfort impacts mobility. Pain-relieving medication affects alertness. Loss of fluids, lying down at length, sudden movement, medication, and/or anxiety can cause dizziness. Gait and balance changes can occur. The nurse uses a fall risk assessment, implements fall precaution measures, and promotes mobility as appropriate. Patient education is vital, covering topics such as calling for help, not getting up without assistance, and being mindful of equipment cords that can cause tripping.

Scope of Practice Related to Procedures

Procedural Nursing Scope of Practice

The perioperative nurse follows the full continuum of the patient's surgical experience. The nurse protects the patient from harm, in particular during the times when the patient cannot speak for themselves due to anesthesia or sedation. Such duties include advocating for the patient, ensuring safe and quality care, and participating in discharge planning needs. The nurse communicates with the patient preoperatively, provides education, gains understanding of patient decisions, confirms consent, and reviews advance directives. During surgery, the nurse expresses the patient's wishes and provides a safe environment. Postoperatively, they provide for a smooth transition of care. Various roles exist for the perioperative nurse (e.g., surgical scrub nurse, moderate sedation registered nurse, registered nurse circulator, registered nurse first assistant) in accordance with individual scopes of practice, advanced training, and certification.

Surgical Scrub Nurse

The surgical scrub nurse is an integral part of the surgical team, specially trained to work inside the sterile field. Primary responsibilities include preparing the operating room for the surgical procedure, handling instruments, communicating with perioperative team members, and advocating for quality of care. Their expertise and knowledge pertain to the surgical field, aseptic technique, and various types of surgical equipment. They are intimately familiar with the surgical instruments and supplies and ensure that equipment is functioning properly.

In this role, the surgical scrub maintains and safeguards the sterile field. The nurse works directly with the surgeon by understanding their needs, anticipating the stages of the procedure, and handing instruments to them. If a complication arises, the surgical scrub nurse supports the surgeon by providing

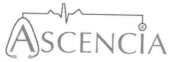

the appropriate instrument or medication. They also communicate with other perioperative team members, including the registered nurse circulator. Importantly, their extensive knowledge of the procedure allows the surgical scrub nurse to be mindful of the patient's safety during surgery.

Moderate Sedation Registered Nurse

The role of the moderate sedation registered nurse is to provide management of the patient receiving moderate sedation, including medication administration in the procedural setting (e.g., endoscopy). In moderate sedation, the patient has a decreased level of consciousness yet is able to respond to verbal commands. The scope of nursing practice is defined by the individual state law and institutional policies, which include competencies required and level of supervision. The nurse must demonstrate competence in the role or attain certification as a certified registered nurse anesthetist (CRNA). Advanced knowledge of perianesthesia and critical care nursing is required, as well as moderate sedation medication administration.

The moderate sedation registered nurse has the primary duty of administering the sedation, monitoring the patient, and reversing the agent as needed. The nurse conducts a pre-sedation assessment to recognize any complications with moderate sedation. This may encompass current medications, medical history, vital signs, cognition, and respiratory status. Responsible for planning the procedure, the nurse prepares the room. During moderate sedation, the nurse has direct patient access and continuously monitors the therapeutic response. Prepared to respond to emergencies, the moderate sedation nurse intervenes urgently to address complications (e.g., compromised airway, oversedation). The nurse oversees the patient recovery from the sedation, conducts a post-procedure assessment, and evaluates the outcome. In addition to moderate sedation, the CRNA may also participate in anesthetic management in the operating room.

Registered Nurse Circulator

Working outside the sterile field, the registered nurse (RN) circulator is accountable for nursing activities that occur throughout the perioperative stages. Their goal is to restore or improve the patient's health from their baseline condition. They support the nursing process by planning and documenting the nursing care through patient assessment, implementation of nursing interventions, and evaluation of outcomes. Preoperatively, the nurse performs an assessment and communicates with the patient to gain an understanding of their particular needs. Because the patient is not aware during surgery, the RN circulator has the important role of patient advocate. The nurse collaborates with the surgical team, oversees the surgical activities, and ensures a safe environment. During emergencies, the RN circulator responds and intervenes as needed. Other responsibilities include providing any additional supplies or equipment. Together with the scrub nurse, the RN circulator can count surgical instruments. Postoperatively, the nurse provides a handoff report to the PACU nurse with the details of the intraoperative events, medications given, and outcomes.

Registered Nurse First Assistant

The registered nurse first assistant (RNFA) is a specially trained nurse who works alongside the surgeon throughout the perioperative phases of care. Role requirements include completion of an RNFA program and a Certified Perioperative Nurse (CNOR) credential. Specific activities are designated by state law and institutional policy. The nurse has a range of responsibilities that encompass the nursing process. Preoperatively, they conduct a nursing assessment, collaborate with the surgical team, and communicate the patient's plan of care. Some RNFAs may write preoperative orders. Intraoperatively, the RNFA supports the surgeon by handling certain surgical instruments, providing surgical site exposure

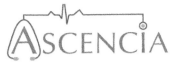

to maintain visibility of the surgical field, and managing the wound. Additionally, they provide hemostasis, which plays a role in controlling surgical bleeding, preserving the patient's physiological functions, and improving patient outcomes. In the postoperative period, the RNFA may write orders, document the intraoperative procedure, provide follow-up care, and participate in discharge planning.

Supplies, Instruments, and Equipment

Surgical team members handling surgical instruments, supplies, and equipment have clinical knowledge for accurate incisions and protecting the staff and patient from injury. Each type of instrument has different variations, shaped and designed according to specific purposes. Some procedures require a heavier tool, while others need an instrument that accommodates finer control when manipulating tissues.

Common surgical instruments are used for cutting and dissection, retracting and gripping tissue, clamping or clipping blood vessels, and suctioning. For cutting and dissecting tissue, examples include the scalpel and scissors. The scalpel creates the skin incision and dissects deeper tissue. Scissors are designed with different traits (e.g., curved or straight, blunt or sharp) to cut and dissect tissue as well as cut dressings and sutures. The tools used for retracting and gripping tissue are the retractor and the dissecting forceps. A retractor holds tissue securely to provide surgical field visibility, locked in place by a ratchet. Dissecting forceps are selected according to size and presence of teeth to grasp and grip tissue.

Clamping instruments serve to occlude blood vessels and constrict tissue. The hemostat controls bleeding by clamping or clipping a vein or artery to provide hemostasis. Different variations are available according to the surgical need, such as clamping a small vessel or a large tissue area. These have an appearance similar to scissorlike pliers, with rings to hold the instrument, a jaw for clamping, and a ratchet for locking the device. Another type of clamping instrument is the vascular clamp, designed to stem blood flow at the surgical site. Suction devices remove blood and other body fluids away from the surgical field. Typically attached to a vacuum source by suction tubing, the equipment is designed according to the quantity of fluid expected.

Other supplies protect the staff and patient to minimize potential harm. The surgical team employs surgical asepsis measures prior to surgery, including a surgical scrub and donning personal protective equipment (PPE). Sponges and brushes are used with antimicrobial agents to scrub the hands and fingernails for 5 minutes. PPE is donned, including a surgical cap, shoe covers, a gown, a mask and goggles (or face shield), and sterile gloves. Surgical drapes serve to create the sterile field to hold the sterile instruments and supplies until needed. Sterile drapes also cover the patient and operating room (OR) table to separate the surgical incision from the surrounding environment. Patient monitors support clinical decision-making to achieve successful outcomes specific to the procedure. General examples include pulse oximetry, capnography, electrocardiogram (ECG), and a noninvasive blood pressure device.

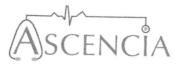

Nutrition

Individualized Nutritional Needs

Malnutrition

Malnutrition is a condition marked by an imbalance of the micronutrients needed to maintain the body's functions. Multiple conditions may lead to malnutrition. These stem from two sources: lack of sufficient nutrients in the diet and malabsorption of the nutrients that are provided. Deficiencies in one or more vitamins or nutrients are a cause of concern that may lead to adverse clinical conditions.

Common vitamin deficiencies include iron, vitamin A, vitamin B complex, vitamin C, magnesium, calcium, potassium, and zinc. Patients may present with hair loss, bleeding gums, weakness, pain, arrhythmias, and neurological disorders such as paresthesias, cognitive impairments, and behavioral issues.

Food allergies have a synergistic effect on the severity of potential nutritional deficiencies. An increase in the number of food allergies an individual has leads to an increase in effects on the body systems. Wheat allergies can lead to a lack of iron, vitamins B6 and B12, folic acid, vitamin D, copper, and zinc absorption.

Celiac disease, an autoimmune disorder caused by a severe reaction to gluten, results in damaging inflammation to the lining of the small intestine. Mucosal damage of the villi severely limits the absorbability of the digestive system. Fat-soluble vitamins and fatty acids cannot be absorbed. Individuals who have celiac disease can become severely iron deficient. Symptoms of celiac disease include diarrhea, steatorrhea, and weight loss. Failure of growth may occur in children.

Avoiding dairy is a primary cause of vitamin D deficiency. This may be due to an allergy, lactose intolerance, or dietary choice. Total avoidance of dairy products causes leaching of calcium from bone for cellular function. This can progress to osteoporosis or osteopenia.

Vomiting and diarrhea, whether due to a medical condition or self-induced, limit the amount of food that reaches the digestive system and the time within the system needed to effectively absorb the nutrients. Anorexia is an eating disorder marked by intentional starvation or excessive caloric burning through compulsive exercise. Another eating disorder that affects consumption and absorption of sufficient micronutrients is bulimia. Bulimia is self-induced purging after binging an excessive amount of calories. Purging may be accomplished via self-induced vomiting, laxative use, or excessive exercise. These types of purging can cause severe electrolyte and nutrient imbalances that may lead to life-threatening dysrhythmias, absent menses, muscle weakness, dry skin, loss of hair, impaired wound healing, and susceptibility to illness.

Socioeconomic factors strongly influence access to food resources. A poor diet may be caused by poverty, lack of access to food, psychological barriers, and limited availability of healthy foods. Nurses may support patients identified with barriers by being knowledgeable of local and national programs that provide resources and funds to improve nutrition for high-risk populations. Populations at most risk include individuals with disabilities, certain racial and ethnic groups, and rural dwellers.

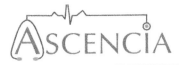

Disease Processes with Dietary Restrictions

The cardiovascular system is composed of circulatory vessels and the heart that work in conjunction to transport blood to the body's organs. This system is sensitive to changes in fluid shifts that can cause overhydration or dehydration. Heart failure is the ineffective pumping action of the heart muscle. This limits the system's ability to effectively transport blood to the organs. A major cause of exacerbation of heart failure is fluid overload. Increased sodium levels have a direct effect on fluid retention, urinary retention, weight gain, and increased thirst, causing increased fluid intake. Excessive sodium consumption, a diet high in saturated and trans fats, and alcohol intake are modifiable risk factors for hypertension. A high-fat diet may lead to hypercholesterolemia, which is a primary factor in the development of plaque formation within the circulatory vessels. This plaque buildup impedes blood flow and can result in critical blockages that cause injury or ischemia to vital organs or extremities. Ischemic cardiac events are life-threatening and require immediate intervention via percutaneous cardiac intervention.

Diabetes mellitus is a metabolic disease where the pancreas is unable to supply the required insulin needed for glucose control. The cells are unable to transport glucose into the cell for energy production. There are two types of diabetes mellitus: type I and type II. Type I is a chronic, life-long disease marked by a complete deficiency or severe insufficiency of insulin production and is usually identified during childhood. Individuals with type I require insulin supplementation to maintain euglycemia. Type II diabetes is two-fold: insulin production does not meet cellular needs, and the cells do not respond, leading to poor uptake. Type II diabetes may not be curable; however, it is possible to manage with a diet that controls blood sugar. This may or may not be in conjunction with insulin or other diabetic medications. It is highly recommended to follow a diet that is high in fiber and low in saturated fats. Simple sugars should be replaced by complex carbohydrates with an increase in the consumption of fresh vegetables and fruits.

The renal system regulates fluid and pH balance through the H+ buffer system and controls electrolyte levels. As protein is broken down, urea, creatine, and ammonia are produced and must be eliminated via the kidney's filtration system. Decreases in kidney function can have widespread detrimental effects, including high blood pressure, hemodynamic instability, and uric crystal buildup. Individuals with kidney dysfunction should be advised to decrease sodium intake to less than approximately 2000 mg daily. To reduce the effects of metabolite buildup from protein breakdown, it is advised to limit and choose lean animal and plant-based proteins such as chicken, fish, eggs, beans, grains, and nuts. Certain electrolytes are more likely to cause issues in individuals with kidney disease. Foods high in phosphorus (grains, meats, beans, nuts, and dark sodas) and potassium (oranges, potatoes, grains, dairy, beans, and nuts) should be regulated.

Physical Impairments

Diseases that affect the muscles and control of facial and throat movements can be a significant barrier to effective chewing and safe swallowing. Any traumatic brain injury, such as a closed-head injury or cerebrovascular accident (CVA), can cause changes to the muscle control of the face, tongue, and throat. With a CVA, a classic sign (facial drooping) may be permanent or take weeks to months to recover movement. The resulting dysphagia puts these patients at a much higher risk for aspiration.

Parkinson's disease results in shaky, spastic movements along with balance and coordination dysfunction. Common medications used to treat this neurological disorder may cause dry mouth as well as mouth and throat pain.

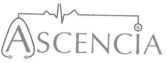

The autoimmune disease multiple sclerosis attacks the myelin sheath protecting nerve fibers. The symptoms caused by this neuromuscular disease vary by individual, often resulting in muscle weakness, paralysis, and impaired function. Swallowing mechanisms may be affected, leading to an increased risk for aspiration. Structural dysphagia may also be due to abnormalities involving the pharynx, esophagus, or oral cavity. This can include head and neck malignancies and subsequent radiation, infection of the throat cavity, and esophageal strictures.

For any new disease process or disorder that affects the mouth, throat, upper airway, or esophagus, a swallow study must be ordered and completed prior to the patient taking any medications or food by mouth. Depending on the facility, the nurse or speech therapist may do the initial test to evaluate the swallowing of different thicknesses and textures. If the patient fails this test, a barium swallow may be completed to diagnose the problem.

Patients with tracheostomies may have barriers to swallowing depending on the insertion site of the stoma. Some trach tubes include a cuff that must be deflated prior to eating. Small bites, thorough chewing, and thickened liquids may all assist with preventing aspiration.

Cultural Food Preferences

There are many religious and cultural norms associated with food preferences or dietary rules. Muslims that adhere to Islam tenets may only consume chicken, lamb, goat, or beef that was halal-raised and butchered. Hindus, making up 79 percent of India's population, are usually lacto-vegetarian, consuming dairy but avoiding fish, meat, poultry, and eggs. Fasting periods are common and may be associated with religious days for both Muslims—such as Islam's Ramadan—and Hindus.

Individuals who follow Jewish law are guided by Kashrut, a set of dietary laws that state which foods may be eaten and how they must be prepared. Foods must be kosher; this includes animals that have cloven hooves and chew cud and seafood with scales and fins. Birds of prey are forbidden. Additionally, dairy and meat must not be eaten together.

Mormons avoid any mind-altering substance. This includes caffeinated beverages, tobacco, alcohol, or illicit drugs.

There are many socio-cultural food practices based on region that include eating patterns and trends, different sources of protein, and characteristics of the meals.

In Mexican families, homemade food is seen as an important tradition and meals are typically eaten as a family. Black beans and steak are commonly eaten proteins. Foods traditionally prepared may be high in fat and sodium. Chinese culture uses food to build relationships with others; food may also be associated with social status. Rice is a large dietary component with lean meats and seafood; however, meals are high in carbohydrates and sodium. Japanese social norms surrounding foods embrace Washoku, a social practice that aligns food with a person's spirit.

It is important to keep in mind that not all individuals from those regions or associated with those cultures necessarily follow the food practices. Ethnic preferences should never be assumed, and the nurse should ask for individual preferences.

Nutrition Administration Modalities

Enteral

Enteral feeding is the administration of nutrition into the gastrointestinal tract. When a patient is unable to tolerate nutrition through the oral route, alternative routes (via tube delivery) are available that may

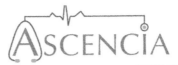

be utilized from one month to a longer term of six months or more. Enteral tube feeding directly bypasses oral intake to deliver to the stomach or lower digestive system.

A tube is inserted through the oral/pharyngeal cavity into the stomach or may be inserted percutaneously into the stomach or small intestine. A nasogastric (NG) tube may be inserted at the bedside by the nurse and does not require special preparation. Once the tube is placed, the nurse should use a large bore syringe to check the pH of the aspirate. Gastric aspirate will show a pH of ≤ 5.5. Auscultating a small air bolus above the epigastric space is common practice but not the gold standard. Best practice indicates that an x-ray should be used to verify appropriate placement. The chest x-ray should show that the NG tube is visualized midline to the level of the diaphragm, that the carina is bisected, the radiopaque tip may be seen below the left hemi diaphragm, and that the placement of the tip is at least 10 centimeters past the gastroesophageal junction. NG tubes should be avoided with long-term use as the breakdown of nares, ulceration, esophageal reflux, and aspiration pneumonia can occur.

Gastrostomy (G), gastrojejunal (GJ), and jejunostomy (J) tubes are typically inserted under fluoroscopy or surgically. These methods create a stoma directly through the abdominal wall into the stomach. A percutaneous endoscopic gastrostomy (PEG) is the preferred option for long-term feeding. This method places the tube via a lighted flexible tube (called an endoscope) that is inserted orally and shines a bright light through the abdominal wall to guide the puncture for stoma formation.

Any enteral nutrition that is delivered directly to the stomach, either via G tube or PEG tube, is digested just as though it were ingested through the oral route. When the tube is advanced further into the jejunum, the stomach is bypassed. For conditions such as atrophic gastritis or gastroparesis, this allows the enteral formula to reach the jejunum. The jejunum primarily functions to absorb fatty acids, amino acids, and glucose. This decreases the risk for aspiration as the feeding tube travels past the pyloric sphincter, preventing regurgitation as the formula is not able to backflow to the stomach. As absorption rates differ within the stomach and the jejunum, all GJ tubes have two ports: one that delivers to the stomach and one that delivers to the jejunum. This allows for venting and medication delivery directly to the stomach and separate delivery of formula to the jejunum.

Three types of formula are available: polymeric, hydrolyzed, and modular. Polymeric formulas are best for individuals who do not have an alteration in digestive processes and readily absorb nutrients. Hydrolyzed formulas contain simple carbohydrates, predigested proteins, and a medium-chain triglyceride oil blend. This predigested version is best for individuals receiving delivery to the lower digestive system or who have an impairment in absorbing nutrients. Modular formulas are unique blends meant to supplement deficiencies in an individual's intake and do not meet all nutritional needs. These are appropriate for patients who have some oral intake, but they are not enough to reach nutritional requirements.

Parenteral

Total parenteral nutrition (TPN) is a nutritional drug that delivers the complete macro- and micronutrients that are required to fulfill the patient's nutritional needs. It is used when a patient's digestive system must be bypassed entirely. Conditions that may require TPN include bowel obstruction, cancer, congenital gastrointestinal malformations, hypercatabolic states, and anticipated periods of time where a status of nothing by mouth (NPO) will be required for greater than seven days, such as sepsis and other high acuity conditions.

TPN is a high-risk medication that must be delivered via central venous access. The content has a high osmolarity that has a detrimental effect on the lining of the peripheral vasculature, leading to an

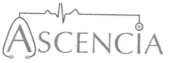

elevated rate of thromboembolism formation. The formula has a high glucose content which may promote bacterial growth. TPN must be refrigerated until the time of administration, and the nurse must employ strict sterile techniques to prevent infection. Specialized tubing with an in-line, 1.2-micron filter is used to prevent patient exposure to pathogens or particulates within the solution. This tubing must be changed every 24 hours to prevent bacterial growth. The delivery system should remain closed, aside from tubing changes. During changes, the patient should be instructed to perform the Valsalva maneuver in order to prevent an air bolus from entering through the central line.

Fluctuations in blood glucose levels are a risk of TPN administration. Blood glucose levels should be closely monitored during the first 36 hours to assess the effect on the patient. Insulin may be added during the pharmaceutical formulation process if the patient continues to be hyperglycemic. Adjustments may be made to the formula should hypoglycemia occur.

The risk for sepsis is extremely high due to central venous access. In addition to sterile technique being utilized with initial access and any line dressing changes, the nurse should assess and monitor the access site for any localized redness, swelling, tenderness, or exudate at the insertion site. An elevated temperature, chills, or rigors must be reported to the attending healthcare provider immediately. Fluid overload may occur if the set rate of administration is too high for the patient's clinical condition. The nurse should monitor for crackles in the lung bases, jugular vein distention, edema, shortness of breath, and hypertension. This risk is elevated for patients who have comorbidities such as congestive heart failure, kidney disease, or liver failure.

Resources for Alternate Nutrition Administration

Interdisciplinary Resources

A patient with dysphagia who will require long-term supplemental nutrition is assigned a primary team to manage the clinical aspects of nutritional support. This typically consists of the attending healthcare provider, an assigned nurse, and a pharmacist. These patients are complex and require additional support or clinical care that may include other departments and specialties. It is not uncommon for these patients to have consultations with a surgical or interventional team and social work, gastroenterology, endocrinology, and mid-level provider specialists. Two key members of the interdisciplinary team specific to dysphagia include the speech therapist and dietician.

Speech Therapist

The speech therapist's initial assessment consists of gathering the patient's medical history, identifying the patient's signs and symptoms of dysphagia, and performing a swallow evaluation to assess swallow function.

The swallow evaluation consists of a trial of different textures and consistencies to identify inconsistencies with mastication and swallowing. The speech therapist will provide the patient with foods such as saltine crackers and document the bites required, the time chewing, and the number of swallows per cracker. Once the patient is finished, they will be asked to speak. Applesauce and liquids in various thickened states may be progressed to, with evaluation of complete swallowing and ability to speak afterward. This evaluation tests for aspiration as gurgles or choking often occurs with verbalization post swallowing. If at any time the patient becomes short of breath, chokes, or is having difficulty talking, the test is immediately aborted. Further evaluation of swallowing may be done through a barium swallow imaging test to diagnose dysphagia.

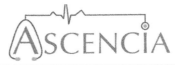

Speech therapists are subject matter experts on assessing and evaluating a patient to determine the severity of dysphagia. Their expertise should be consulted with any patient who is identified as having dysphagia or an increased risk of aspiration. Swallow screening tools, such as the 10-Item Eating Assessment, are readily available for initial use by nursing personnel to determine whether a speech therapy consultation is appropriate. During swallow screening, red flags that indicate that a referral is appropriate include a history of coughing while eating, choking, difficulty swallowing, or drooling. Patients who have disease processes that affect mouth or tongue movement are more prone to difficulties with eating and drinking and should be checked for complete swallowing while eating. Food that remains tucked between the cheeks and gums or under the tongue after swallowing is referred to as pocketing and is a primary aspiration risk.

Dietician

A dietician's role is to provide nutritional screening and assessments to patients who are at high risk for imbalanced nutrition. The dietician must determine the patient's calorie expenditure each day. This is based on three elements: the amount of physical activity, basal energy use, and the thermal feeding effect. The latter is the amount of energy that is required in the digestion and processing of food. Another method used also considers factors such as injury or fever, which increase metabolic catabolism and thereby increase caloric needs. Dieticians are also relied upon by providers to establish a diet and food plan that aligns with dietary and cultural preferences, allergies, and clinical disease processes that require restrictions.

During hospitalization, a patient may be identified as a good candidate for further education or management of dietary needs in an inpatient or outpatient setting. The dietician is a resource for managing dietary restrictions, giving suggestions and education on how to incorporate a variety of food sources to improve nutrition, and arranging and following up on any parenteral or enteral feedings that will need to be continued post-discharge. Patients who are identified with nutritional imbalances, are obese, are underweight, or have other dietary or wellness needs that may be difficult for the patient or family to fulfill may be advised of resources within the community.

Indications for Alternate Nutrition Administration

Enteral

Dysphagia may occur with any pathophysiological process that affects swallowing. This results in the inability of food, liquid, or medications to pass through the upper gastrointestinal tract unimpeded. There are four stages to swallowing that involve nerve, muscle, and neurological interaction to successfully occur. The oral preparation stage begins when food is chewed and mixed with saliva to begin the enzymatic breakdown process. A food bolus or liquid is moved towards the back of the throat by the tongue. Voluntarily, swallowing starts when the food enters the pharynx in the pharyngeal stage. Once past the epiglottis, involuntary control pushes the food or liquid further along as the throat relaxes and the epiglottis closes. Gravity moves liquids through the esophagus via gravity while the bolus is moved along by undulating reflex movements towards the stomach. When swallowing occurs, the lower esophageal sphincter opens, allowing food and drink to pass. Failure at any stage leads to abnormal passage of food or drink.

Upper gastrointestinal dysfunction that may require enteral feedings involves an alteration in the normal passage of chyme (gastric juice combined with partially digested food) or a dysfunction or inflammation in the lining of the digestive tract preventing the absorption of nutrients. These disorders include Crohn's disease, bowel obstruction, ulcerative colitis, or gastroparesis.

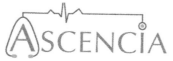

The risk for malnutrition is elevated in hospitalized individuals, and it can lead to poor outcomes, impaired healing, and increased morbidity and mortality. When metabolic requirements exceed the amount of nutritional intake, the risk for infection, apathy, depression, and postoperative complications increases. Enteral nutritional intake aims to deliver sufficient nutrients to improve patient outcomes. For enteral nutrition to be effective, the gastrointestinal tract must be accessible and functioning. Patients that are appropriate to be considered for enteral nutrition include those with upper GI dysfunction with gastric function remaining intact.

Critical care patients who are unable to ingest food (including comatose patients, patients with a TBI, or stroke patients) are ideal candidates. Patients with disorders or disease processes that prevent the sufficient intake of calories, such as people with anorexia or those undergoing treatment for cancer, may benefit from having nutrition delivered via the enteral route.

Parenteral

TPN is an effective alternative when enteral feedings are contraindicated; however, this is the least cost-effective and most complicated method of providing total nutrition. Several factors must be considered, including a robust conversation with the patient and family regarding the risks versus benefits of this alternative form of nutrition. As the digestive system is completely bypassed, this route of nutrition is necessary for patients who do not have intact gastrointestinal function. A lack of gastrointestinal function may stem from dysphagia, loss of functional movement through the digestive system, or intestinal malabsorption leading to nutritional deficiencies.

Bowel rest is effective for treating inflammatory intestinal diseases such as Crohn's disease or ulcerative colitis. Bypassing the digestive route and delivering caloric and nutrient intake directly into the bloodstream reduces stimulation of intestinal mucosa.

TPN may be required for patients who have undergone massive bowel resections or have had a loss of function in a major segment of the bowel. Short bowel syndrome occurs when the amount of functional intestinal tract is insufficient to maintain nutrient absorption. The length of the functional small bowel dictates TPN requirements and the length of time typically needed. Patients who have less than 60 centimeters may need TPN for the remainder of their life. Patients who have between 90 and 180 centimeters usually require supplementation for less than one year.

TPN is also used when enteral feedings are not appropriate. Absolute contraindications to enteral feedings include bowel obstruction, severe or prolonged ileus, active gastrointestinal bleeding, and mesenteric ischemia. Attempting an enteral feeding in this patient population may result in further complications, including increased obstruction of the bowel and intestinal perforation. Ulceration, abscess, bleeding, and pancreatitis may follow. Patients' hemodynamic stability may be compromised with hypotensive or hypovolemic shock, peritonitis, and sepsis related to small bowel necrosis.

Holistic Patient Care

Patient-Centered Care

Patient-Centered Care

Effective Communication

One of the most important aspects of developing a connection with a patient is done through communication. This can be verbal and nonverbal. The focus of patient-centered care is to put the patient at the center of the care team. This involves building a friendly rapport and establishing trust through engaging and showing interest in the patient's experiences, history, and current concerns. Verbal communication is a method of conveying and receiving information via spoken and written words. The most important aspect of communication is that the receiver interprets the message as the sender intended. Understanding is key to effective communication.

Nonverbal communication is just as important in building a strong clinical relationship with the patient. Any barriers must be identified and corrected. Healthcare providers should be aware of their body language and presentation. Unless culturally inappropriate, the provider should face the patient and maintain good eye contact without appearing to stare. Being at the same level as the patient, whether standing or sitting, can prevent the patient from feeling intimidated. The arms should be held naturally to the side or with palms facing forward. Crossing of the arms should be avoided as this presents a threatening stance. Facial expressions should be friendly and relaxed.

Communication can take many mediums and may be done face-to-face, via telephone, or by video conference. Consideration should be taken regarding the patient's preferences and culture, tone and volume of voice, the volume level and privacy of the area, and potential language barriers. An interpreter may be required if the patient's primary language is not English or if they require an assistive device for hearing or visual deficits.

Each participant in a conversation is responsible for engaging via active listening. Key elements of active listening include using body language to show that the provider is listening and providing affirmation that the meaning is understood or requires further details. Stating "yes" or "can you tell me more about this" encourages the patient to continue. Feedback is important to acquire; this can be accomplished through open-ended questions and clarification. Judgment should be held back, along with minimal interruptions to the patient's discussion. Once the patient is finished talking, any opinion given in response should be delivered respectfully.

Interacting with healthcare professionals and having concerns over personal health events can be a stressful situation for the patient. Being open to listening and understanding a patient's experiences and sharing their fears, victories, and emotions can help alleviate that stress. Showing empathy and conveying trust shows that the nurse or provider is giving the patient their full attention, that their concerns are being listened to, and that their best interests are being taken seriously. This can alleviate patient fears and open the way to a two-way conversation that builds the patient relationship with respect, while also meeting the patient's needs. Research has shown that establishing patient-centered

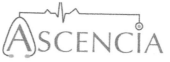

communication increases safety, patient satisfaction, and the use of community resources, and it improves the overall social support network.

Patient and Family Involvement

A meaningful care plan considers the lifestyle, needs, and personal preferences of the patient. Patient-centered care supports the active involvement of the patient and family with treatment options; creating mutually established goals; and informing the patient of the type, timing, and medical providers involved with interventions. Finally, the patient will be actively involved with how goals and outcomes are being evaluated, be active in reporting signs and symptoms, and be able to identify positive and negative changes related to interventions and changes to the treatment plan.

Sharing information with the family may be accomplished with bedside reports and provider rounds that take place with the patient and family present. Incorporating the patient and family into updates and discussions of the care plan provides an opportunity for questions and clarifications from the clinical care providers. Additionally, the patient and family should be encouraged to participate in skilled nursing care, physical therapy, and completion of activities of daily living early in the hospitalization. Each time medications are administered, it is advisable for the nurse to discuss the medication and what it is for. This helps to facilitate a timely and safe discharge, as the patient and family are familiar with the care being provided and how that may be accommodated past the hospitalization. This can also be an opportunity for the nurse to assess the feasibility of the patient and family managing care in the home environment. This is also an opportunity for the nurse to request a social work consult early on if it appears that home care would not be appropriate or if a higher level of care is warranted prior to home discharge.

Patient Advocacy

As the care provider who spends a significant amount of time with the patient, the nurse's role in advocacy is paramount to a patient's outcome. Advocacy in healthcare is the act of upholding beneficence, promoting equality, and retaining a person's dignity and rights. Nurses have an opportunity to uphold advocacy by identifying barriers, disparities, and gaps in care based on the patient's individual circumstances. These factors may include educational level, interpreter needs for native languages, cultural preferences, financial or insurance concerns, and transportation impediments.

At the bedside, nurses are most often called upon to uphold advocacy by ensuring the patient's concerns are addressed and their voice is heard by the healthcare team. The nurse may assist the patient in translating medical terms and explaining the care plan in a way that is meaningful and understandable. Complex diagnoses, treatments, and outcomes are difficult for many people who are not familiar with the healthcare field. The nurse may provide education and resources, ensure that referrals are complete, and provide guidance on optimizing health outcomes.

Nurses should be abreast of best practice for their field of expertise. This may be accomplished through attending conferences and reading evidence-based practice literature on the most common patient diagnoses and treatments that are within the area of care that is provided. Nursing journal articles are a great resource for learning best practice and innovative methods to provide care. Nurses may also choose to continue their education. An advanced degree allows a nurse to practice at a higher scope, leading to increased opportunities for individual, community, and national advocacy. Opportunities to lead at a national level may be found in political and governmental policy development and change.

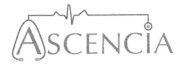

Patient Satisfaction Management

Patient Surveys

Patient experiences may be discovered via accreditation body surveys, patient feedback, quality reviews post-close calls, adverse or sentinel events, and leadership rounding. A facility may opt-in to participate in consultative and watchdog data collection to be disseminated in identifying patient care areas that have deficits or opportunities for improvement.

This data can guide an organization's mission statement, culture, future developments, and care service lines. Opportunities for improvement that are identified may lead to improved access and quality of care within a community. Many organizations focus on improving patient safety with a focus on finding system errors that may be corrected to prevent recurrence. High scores in patient satisfaction, safety, and quality can be a motivation for patients to choose that facility for their care.

The Hospital Consumer Assessment of Healthcare Providers and Systems (HCAHPS) survey evaluates a patient's perception of the quality of their hospital stay. Categories include the environment's cleanliness, the likelihood to recommend the facility to others, provider and care team communication, management of care and transitions, medication knowledge, and discharge understanding.

Complaints and Grievances

When a patient or patient's family believes that the patient's rights have been or are being violated, a complaint may be submitted to the facility. Each facility has a chain of command for complaints based on the type and severity. A Patient Advocate, Patient Representative, or similar team may be employed by the organization to facilitate resolutions of complaints.

Complaints most often seen in healthcare include delays in care, lack of empathy, not being included in care plan development, poor communication, ambiguous diagnosis, inappropriate provider bedside manner, and breach of patient confidentiality. Discussing the patient's expectations and setting reasonable goals can assist in mitigating complaints.

Any complaints voiced to the healthcare team should be taken seriously. These should be brought to the nurse manager's attention to be addressed through the appropriate chain of command. Complaints may be formal or informal and may involve an easy-to-solve matter or an issue that is much more complicated. Matters that can be resolved in the moment or within 24 hours are considered informal and, as such, do not require significant documentation or follow-up. More serious complaints require significant attention and should be referred to the quality and patient safety department. This fulfills a federally regulated process that is required for hospitals accredited by The Joint Commission and creates a log for addressing the problem and providing solutions to prevent future occurrences.

A grievance is a formal type of complaint that is usually of a more serious nature. This could include a poor patient outcome, injury, egregious care, or lack of respect for the patient's concerns and needs. These may be filed to the administrative department of the facility or to an accrediting body, such as the Centers for Medicare and Medicaid Services or The Joint Commission. Grievances are more likely to be investigated and can progress to litigation should the patient or family not feel that the outcome is satisfactory.

Service Recovery

Complaints should be directed to the facility's patient experience or advocacy team. They are skilled in providing unbiased, empathetic communication aimed at exploring the patient's issue, meeting with the

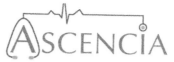

care team involved, and developing a remedy that is satisfactory to the patient. The patient should be followed up with during their hospitalization to assess whether actions remedied the complaint. Another follow-up may be appropriate post-discharge, depending on the type and severity of complaint, especially if it involves a gap in care, egregious behavior, medical mistakes, or misconduct.

When a patient complaint or grievance involves a system's error or process that needs to be improved, the facility must take steps to rectify the root cause of the matter. A peer review is often employed to investigate the validity, factors, and cause of the complaint. Interviews of care providers involved, the patient, and the patient's family are completed in order to provide a comprehensive picture of the issue at hand. Facilities may implement a method of capturing complaints and grievances so that they may be analyzed and addressed. A grievance committee is assistive in the review process. When the system's issues are identified, it is advantageous to adjust policies, procedures, and training to accommodate for change that improves patient satisfaction and safety.

Adopting a proactive stance to reduce the probability of patient complaints is found to be very effective. This can be done by employing strategies aimed at addressing a patient's needs before they become concerns or complaints. Training bedside and frontline staff to be effective at listening and responding to patient concerns is a culture change that can drive forward patient safety and satisfaction. Provider and staff training should include effective communication techniques, such as empathy and active listening. Additionally, a specialized team may be formed that has training to deal with and provide solutions to issues prior to escalation.

Service recovery is an adjunctive method for providing the patient with a reasonable reparation for their complaint or grievance. This is supplemental to attempts to rectify the problem. At times, even when complaints are resolved, the patient may still feel that they have not had fair or just treatment or care. Using service recovery is a method of improving the patient relationship and regaining trust. Recovery may come in the form of gift cards, free parking passes, meal tickets, or reductions in charges.

Diversity and Inclusion

Cultural and Linguistic Needs and Resources

There is a wide variety and ever-changing population of patients that are seen in the healthcare setting. It is important to provide the necessary resources and tools to break down language barriers. The most common language barrier occurs when the healthcare provider and patient do not share a native language. This can lead to healthcare disparities and further disproportion already disadvantaged groups. Risk assessments may identify gaps in care and determine the need for readily available educational materials in languages that are prevalent in specific care settings. In addition, foreign language translation services must be established with providers and healthcare staff trained on their use within clinical settings. Providing these services increases access to care, improves patient safety, and prevents medical errors due to misunderstanding. To prepare for the need for interpretive services, scheduling and screening staff should inquire about the patient's preferred language and any other preferences they may have regarding educational materials and communication.

When a patient has a sensory impairment, such as blindness or deafness, alternative communication formats can improve comprehension of healthcare literature, increase communication, and provide a fuller understanding of their individual healthcare condition. Healthcare facilities should have sign language services in the same way that foreign language interpretation is provided. Braille is invaluable

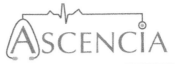

to individuals who are blind or have significant vision loss. Large print and specialized audio formats are other alternative communication methods to incorporate into communication and educational materials.

For non-verbal, cognitively impaired, or low-literacy learners, pictures and symbols may be an appropriate means of enhancing communication. A commonly used tool that utilizes pictures is the Wong-Baker FACES Pain Rating Scale. The tool may be used for a wide range of audiences, from three years of age and up. Communication boards with easy-to-understand words and illustrations may prove ideal for addressing patient needs, signs and symptoms, and requests.

Staff and healthcare providers who are bilingual can be a great asset to an organization. Having a diverse staff with knowledge and fluency in another language and culture encourages acceptance and inclusivity. Patients who recognize their own culture and language as being represented are more likely to establish trust with their providers and the healthcare system. Further, promoting competent leaders who represent the diversity of their communities is an essential component in promoting a just and equitable culture.

Executive leadership establishes the forward momentum and vision of an organization. C-suite leadership should ideally be a cross-sectional archetype of the communities that are served. Often, this is far from the reality of seats at the table, and a focus on promoting inclusivity must be considered in the selection process. Bringing a more rounded perspective to leadership at the top-level for decision-making processes can increase the ability to adapt to personalized, patient-centered care; improve communication that is centered on providing access and inclusivity to the demographics of the area; expand targeted care to underrepresented groups; and adapt to identified gaps in patient care.

Creating an atmosphere that embraces cultural competence requires the support of leadership to develop policies and procedures that offer education, training, and opportunities to expand services that support diversity and inclusivity. Several states mandate that healthcare provider continued education include a component of inclusivity, equity, and inclusion training.

Other methods to promote diversity in the healthcare workplace include promoting inclusive hiring practices via actively seeking candidates with diverse backgrounds, encouraging equity in pay, providing in-house diversity and inclusivity committees and programs, offering equal opportunities for career and personal development, listening and responding to feedback regarding bias and discrimination, and creating teams that are diverse and indiscriminate.

Implicit Bias

Subconscious bias, also known as implicit bias, relates to the attitudes and stereotypes that are carried unconsciously and have a profound effect on actions, decisions, and beliefs. These may not necessarily be negative but do influence the decision-making process in a way that may not be based on reality. Social behavior is driven by our understanding of the world through our experiences, but these may not reflect an accurate representation of events or ideals. Individuals may be completely unaware that they carry implicit biases, but these do predict behaviors. These may have strong influences on beliefs and judgments of race, gender, socioeconomic status, and many other labels in society.

Implicit bias, even when it is a positive assumption, is destructive to promoting and building an equitable, diverse, and culturally competent organization. Allowing bias within healthcare providers can lead to healthcare disparities among patients and fellow healthcare workers.

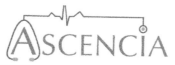

Cultural competence training must address implicit bias because it is largely underrecognized and underrepresented due to its pervasiveness and latency. Training should focus on understanding the implicit bias that is within an organization at both a macro and micro level. The racial perceptions that employees have may be evaluated through investigation of reports of unfair practices and claims of discrimination. Leadership may seek to identify established norms that are prevalent within care units and departments. From these identified biases, comprehensive training may be developed that ensures these issues are addressed. Interactive education that encourages participants to delve into and consider the experiences in their lives that may have built their own implicit biases can be very effective in breaking down the barriers toward an inclusive and equitable workforce. Building policies and procedures that align with training promotes an ongoing commitment to combating implicit bias. Ongoing training may build upon the initial recognition and acknowledgment to build the skills and knowledge needed to prevent biases from having detrimental effects on patient care and employee engagement. It is most effective when the training continues to address self-evaluation of implicit biases, provides strategies to encourage emotional intelligence, and promotes team building.

Health Promotion and Education for Patients and Families

Health Maintenance and Disease Prevention

Promoting simple health practices that research has shown to improve overall well-being and longevity is an important part of patient teaching. Self-care plays a large role in a patient's health status and overall quality of life.

Increased activity has been shown to improve cardiac function, reduce insulin resistance, maintain euglycemia, reduce arthritic and joint pain, and maintain weight control. Aerobic activity of thirty minutes a day for five days each week may also improve neurological function. It is suggested that this level of exercise has the potential to improve cognitive function and retain memory, reasoning, and judgment, thereby reducing the progression of dementia.

The 2020–2025 dietary guidelines promoted by the Centers for Disease Control focus on incorporating a variety of healthy food choices into the daily meal plan. Vegetables, fruits, whole grains, and fat-free or low-fat milk and milk product options are important to reap full health benefits. Vegetables and fruits provide the most nutrients when a wide variety of colors are chosen. Protein should include lean meats, poultry, and seafood. Vegetarian options include legumes such as peas, beans, soy-based foods, seeds, and nuts.

Ensuring that the body is properly hydrated has many health benefits. Dehydration may lead to forgetfulness, fatigue, headache, fever, constipation, and kidney stone formation. Severe dehydration may cause seizures, kidney failure, shock, coma, and death. On average, public health sources recommend that an adequate daily fluid intake is approximately 100 ounces for men and 70 ounces for women.

Eating a healthy diet and maintaining weight within a healthy range can stave off many diseases including diabetes, cardiovascular diseases, and cholecystitis. Obesity is also linked to a higher mortality

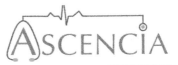

rate, increased stroke risk, earlier progression of osteoarthritic changes, sleep apnea, and mental illness—including anxiety, clinical depression, and other mental afflictions.

In addition to a healthy diet, cardiac diseases are highly sensitive to fluid shifts that may be caused by sodium consumption. It is suggested that individuals with mild cardiac disease limit salt intake to less than 3000 milligrams per day. Individuals with moderate to severe heart failure should restrict consumption further and ensure that no more than 2000 milligrams are included in their daily intake.

Lung diseases are exacerbated by smoking. Refraining from tobacco and marijuana consumption can reduce the increased risk or flare-ups of established respiratory diseases such as asthma, COPD, and emphysema. Avoiding going outside when the air quality is poor or when pollen levels are high can prevent further respiratory distress.

Health Literacy and Teaching Methods

For a patient to be a fully contributing partner in the healthcare team, personal health literacy is an essential skill that can be made easier by the healthcare team. Assessing a patient's educational level, preferred language, and the best way to learn should be the initial conversation with any patient. The healthcare team must adapt to the patient's needs to truly embrace a patient-centered relationship.

Nurse navigators and coordinators are components of a relatively new concept that has been established in many organizations to assist patients with the complex relationship of clinical care, medication management, symptom progression, and alignment of resources to meet the patient's needs. The goal is to provide the patient with the knowledge, tools, and abilities to effectively understand their healthcare plan, be an active partner within the healthcare team, and evaluate the patient's knowledge and working skills to follow the care plan. With continued assessment of the patient's ability to follow the advice of the healthcare team and the response to ordered treatments, adjustments to the treatment direction may be made to enhance the patient's health and quality of life.

Health illiteracy can have many detrimental effects on a patient's care and understanding of their diagnoses and well-being. This includes receiving delayed treatment, medication errors, poor health outcomes, and requiring increased treatment length or the need for additional treatment. Rather than preventive measures, delayed treatment and care leads to disease progression.

There are strategies that nurses and the care team may incorporate to assist patients with improving their health literacy and autonomy over their own health. Time should be made for the patient to receive sufficient education in an environment that is safe, uninterrupted, and allows for easy conversation. Polls have suggested that patients often feel uncomfortable asking questions or inquiring about other concerns when the environment is not welcoming.

Printed material that is at a level of middle-school reading is most effective for reaching a broad audience. Making use of illustrations with simple, clear statements that are incorporated into easy-to-carry handouts, such as pamphlets, allows a patient to take the information with them. This can enhance discussion with family or other individuals involved in the patient's care.

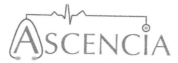

Palliative/End-of-Life Care

Palliative or End-of-Life Patient/Caregiver Resources

Palliative vs. Hospice Care

When an individual experiences a debilitative, progressive disease or is at end-of-life, the goal of care is to provide comfort, relieve pain, and maintain the patient's dignity while managing their symptoms. This may be achieved through palliative care or hospice care, depending on the patient's condition, expected lifespan, and goals of treatment. There is a distinct difference between these two care avenues. Palliative care is designed to provide alleviation with curative measures along with treatment goals aimed at improving daily living. In contrast, hospice care is geared toward providing comfort when death is imminent and does not contain the component of providing treatment that will improve or cure the patient's condition.

Palliative care is most often used for disease processes that are chronic and have a debilitating effect on the patient's quality of life. These may include heart failure, cancer, end-stage renal failure, neurodegenerative disease, or severe respiratory diseases such as COPD and emphysema. There is no limitation on the type of treatment, and it may include curative medications or procedures. Other invasive procedures (such as debulking cancerous tumors) may be aimed more towards alleviating symptoms of pain or discomfort rather than curing. A holistic, integrated care team is employed to manage the patient's well-being and spiritual, social, nutritional, and lifestyle needs. The palliative care team may include providers from specialty services such as cardiology, oncology, and rheumatology in addition to a palliative care specialist. Other members of the team include nurses, nutritionists, social workers, and chaplains.

Hospice care does provide a holistic and comprehensive approach to care aimed at alleviating pain and discomfort; however, the patient's condition has been deemed incurable and is at the end-of-life stage. At this point, all curative measures have been exhausted and the patient's condition continues to decline. Hospice care may begin when a provider declares that a patient with a terminal illness has six months or less to live if the disease process continues a natural progression. The hospice team consists of providers specialized in hospice care and pain management, nurses, social workers, chaplain or spiritual counselors, and volunteer services. The patient and family may choose to have care provided in the home with arrangements to have visiting providers and on-call assistance to provide 24-hour access to resources. Care may also be provided in a hospice care center that is staffed and provides live-in care services.

Physical Care

In palliative and end-of-life care, pain relief therapy is a focal intervention. As with standard pain guidelines, a multi-modal approach is taken. Non-medicinal approaches such as guided imagery, warm blankets, massage, and music therapy may provide adjunctive relief in addition to drug therapy. Analgesic medication may start with NSAIDs and increase to low-dose opioids, dependent upon the patient's previous drug regimen and tolerance to opioids. When pain remains unrelieved, stronger forms of medicinal pain management may be considered. Strong opioids—such as morphine, hydromorphone, and fentanyl—are utilized to treat intractable pain that remains unrelieved with standard treatment.

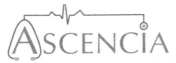

Shortness of breath that may be caused by a disease process affecting the lungs, a tumor that prevents lung expansion, or dyspnea induced by the supply-and-demand mismatch is a phenomenon experienced by 90 percent of patients during their last three days of life. Air hunger, regardless of cause, can be very uncomfortable and is appropriately treated with oxygen supplementation for both palliative and hospice patients. Opioids have also been found to be effective in treating dyspnea in the terminal patient by reducing the respiratory drive. Respiratory secretions that cannot be cleared effectively may also cause shortness of breath. Suctioning and encouraging fluids may help. Medications that dry secretions, such as antimuscarinics, are helpful in managing saliva production.

Cachexia, severe weight loss, and malnutrition are complications of progressive diseases, especially cancers. The body's metabolism is raised to compensate for the energy expenditure used by the exponential cell growth of cancer and cardiorespiratory demand. Combined with poor appetite, nausea, and gastrointestinal distress, patients are often unable to intake the amount of calories needed to maintain their weight. There are certain medications that may help stimulate appetite. Additional calories may be administered via enteral or parenteral nutrition.

Terminal agitation may occur during end-of-life care due to chronic discomfort. This may exhibit itself as behaviors such as aimlessness, labile emotions, and a short attention span. This is similar to delirium, and the patient may present as having hyperactive, hypoactive, or mixed responses to stimulus. This may be caused by certain medications, such as opioids and chemotherapy. Other causes include inadequate pain management, organ failure, and hypoxemia.

Spiritual and Cultural Care

Palliative and hospice care should strive to include a component of spirituality that is individualized and meaningful to the patient's needs. The spiritual needs of the patient may be diverse with preferences for ritual and culture. Patient preferences should be identified upon establishment of the care plan. Acknowledging spiritual requests and accommodating preferred methods of prayer or ceremony have positive effects on the patient's daily life. Patients with chronic, debilitating diseases or those nearing end-of-life report struggles such as fear of suffering, pain, feelings of despair, issues with body image, and longing for the past. Incorporating the patient's spiritual preferences into care and providing opportunities for the patient to participate in their preferred way can improve their feelings towards hope, coping, belonging, having purpose and meaning, and strengthening their faith. Spirituality and cultural customs may play a significant role in how a patient approaches decision-making. Advocating for these preferences to be respected and adhered to by the palliative or hospice care team can improve the quality of life, decrease depressive symptoms, and lessen anxiety and distress about the concept of death.

There are many ways a patient may wish to partake in spiritual and religious rituals or rites that may be performed within the patient's home or care center. These may be individual or include family and friends. Certain religions, such as Catholicism, may have a representative of the faith that will visit the patient and perform a rite, such as reading the Last Rites. Native American patients may request a shaman and perform a smudging ceremony. Other forms of rituals can include reading from a sacred text, chanting, praying, playing music, burning incense, and meditating. At the end of life, patients often experience a desire to express meaning in their lives. Spiritual and cultural requests can help a patient reconnect with their life, give an understanding of what their life has meant, express how they would like to be remembered, and seek or give forgiveness. Sharing their life story can provide the patient with a profound sense of peace and acceptance of their circumstances.

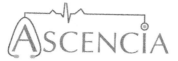

Caregiver Resources

The primary caregiver and family involved with the care of a patient who has a severe illness or is in hospice are involved in an extremely stressful and life-altering situation. The nurse and care team may hold a meeting with the caregiver and family to assess their needs and ability to cope.

There can be significant emotional and physical strain on a caregiver due to being awakened at night; assisting with daily living needs (including physically demanding tasks such as ambulation, toileting, and positioning); and disruptions in family routines, career, and social life. This can lead to the family and caregiver feeling trapped or impeded from participating fully in life and may subsequently lead to feelings of guilt, depression, burnout, resentment, and hopelessness.

The care team should include a social worker to evaluate the socioeconomic status of the caregiver and patient and assess if any resources are needed. Caring for a family member, whether in a part-time or full-time capacity (or if the patient has opted to be admitted to a facility for palliative or hospice care) can be a significant financial burden.

As the patient's disease progresses or is at the point of end-of-life, the family may be dealing with grief in anticipation of death. Resources available for caregiver and family support include support groups aimed at helping caregivers, grief counselors, organizations that represent the specific disease or disability of the patient, and church or religious groups. Hospice benefits provide counseling services, chaplains or spiritual counselors, and volunteer services.

End-of-Life Preferences

Advance Directives

Advance directives in healthcare are legal documents that declare the patient's medical and health objectives for care when they become unable to communicate; these may delegate an individual to make decisions on behalf of the patient in certain circumstances. There are three main types of advance directives: the living will, durable power of attorney (POA), and healthcare proxy. Rules for these legal documents differ between states, and the counsel understands the legally binding capability of each document. These documents may need to be signed and notarized to be legally binding.

The living will is a written document that communicates to the healthcare team what treatments the patient elects in the case of an emergency in which the patient cannot make their own decisions. This occurs when a healthcare provider determines that the patient is incapacitated due to a cognitive process, terminal illness, or coma.

A healthcare proxy is an advance directive where the patient chooses another person to act as an agent when unable to make their own decisions. This surrogate or representative is entrusted by the patient to act on behalf of and advocate for the patient's rights, values, and wishes. When creating this document, state rules should be reviewed to ensure that the proxy meets the requirements to be a healthcare agent. This individual should not be a healthcare professional who is part of the medical care team due to potential ethical conflicts. Commonly, an immediate family member such as a spouse, adult child, or sibling is assigned this role, but it may be another trusted member of the patient's social circle—such as a friend or member of a faith community.

The POA is a similar document to the healthcare proxy; however, this agent is authorized to make financial decisions on behalf of the patient.

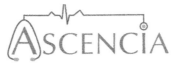

Nurses experience the dilemma of patients who have not created advance directives when a crisis occurs, creating confusion and leaving the family to attempt to decide for the patient. Having conversations early on with the patient about the options that are available to delineate wishes in a clear and concise manner can alleviate the concern and burden upon the patient and family if the patient becomes incapacitated. Often this information is requested upon admission to a procedure or hospitalization and documented in the patient's chart. If the patient does not have a legal document drafted, many healthcare organizations have advance directive forms for the patient to complete and have notarized on-site. The nurse should familiarize themselves with these documents, be able to answer questions regarding the purpose of the forms, and assist with explaining the options a patient may elect. The nurse should also familiarize themselves with state and organizational guidelines regarding next of kin.

Code Status

Code status is a healthcare provider order that directs life-sustaining treatment. There are three main levels of code status. These options should be detailed in length by the healthcare team prior to the patient making a fully informed decision. Full code indicates that all resuscitative measures should be taken should the patient have a cardiogenic or pulmonary arrest. These measures include cardiopulmonary resuscitation (CPR) which may include assisted breathing via intubation and mechanical ventilation, defibrillation, and chest compressions. Vasoactive medications may also be administered based on advanced life care support guidelines.

Do not resuscitate (DNR) indicates that in the case of a patient having a pulseless cardiac arrest, all resuscitative measures, including CPR, vasoactive medications, and intubation will not be attempted. The process causing the arrest is allowed to progress until death occurs. DNR is typically reserved for individuals who have an underlying severe or terminal disease.

Do not intubate (DNI) indicates that in the event of a respiratory arrest, there will be no attempts to intubate the patient, but other lifesaving measures may be attempted.

Advance directives are able to communicate very specific instructions related to code status. This can include a full code status with directions to withhold certain care that would normally be administered. An example of this would be for a patient to remain as a full code but not be administered any artificial nutrition. Another example of this type of stipulation would be that a patient may not wish to receive any blood products for personal, ethical, or religious reasons but would want every other measure taken.

Another option is to elect to implement a limited code status. In this case, the patient is able to choose the resuscitative efforts from the healthcare team that they want to have occur and withhold those that conflict with their wishes. This is typically ordered as a DNR that states that certain actions indicated on the form not be taken. Options of care to withhold may include antiarrhythmic drugs, vasoactive medications, defibrillation/cardioversion, chest compressions, mechanical ventilation via mask or endotracheal intubation, and other CPR measures.

Post-Mortem Care

The nurse assigned to the patient will be responsible for the post-mortem care upon the patient's death. While the patient may not have immediate care needs, this is a timely and sensitive period that requires prompt action to ensure optimal outcomes. The body undergoes physical changes due to tissue ischemia, loss of body temperature, and ceasing of circulation. Rigor mortis (stiffening of the body) and livor mortis (purple discoloration) can begin to set in within a short period of time. The nurse must

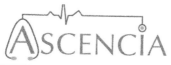

ensure that the body is placed in a supine position with the head of the bed elevated. A fresh pillow should be placed under the patient's head. The family may want to see the patient immediately after death, and this may be accommodated prior to post-mortem care. A quiet and private room should be arranged for the family to wait in while completing post-mortem care.

While performing post-mortem care, standard precautions are followed along with adherence to any special precautions (contact, airborne, etc.) that were in place prior to death. Two patient identifiers are used to confirm the correct patient, and the body is tagged per organization policy. If an autopsy is to be performed, all invasive and indwelling lines must be left in place. Otherwise, remove any indwelling devices such as urinary catheters or endotracheal tubes per policy guidelines. Follow facility policy for the removal of IV and central lines. If the patient has dentures that are not in place, these should be reinserted to improve facial appearance. A rolled towel placed underneath the chin will keep the mouth from remaining open during rigor mortis. The body is washed, any dressings are removed and redressed, and a clean gown is donned. An absorbent pad should be placed under the patient. The family may have a preference for which personal items, such as jewelry, should stay on the patient's body. If anything is removed and given to the family, this should be documented in the patient's chart. Prior to the family returning to view the body, a clean sheet should be placed over the patient.

Grief of Caregiver/Family and the Nurse

As nurses spend a significant time at the bedside, they develop close relationships with the patient and family. The death of the patient is an abrupt loss for all individuals involved in the patient's care. When a patient passes during a nurse's shift, the nurse may go through a gamut of emotions while delivering support to the family and providing post-mortem care to the patient. Nurses can feel responsible for the patient's death, even when expected. Feelings of anxiety, anguish, grief, and sadness are commonly reported.

A supportive organizational culture empowers nurse well-being during this difficult and stressful stage. Some nursing units and organizations may develop practices such as a debriefing, a moment of silence, and buddy programs to assist the primary nurse with completing post-mortem care and tasks. These activities offer comfort and support to the nurse coping with the loss of a patient.

The grieving process after a patient dies can be complicated and last for days to months for both the family and the nurse. Burnout and depression can quickly develop when coping strategies and resources of support are not utilized. There are many online resources and support groups that families or healthcare providers may turn to for support. An internet search for bereavement and grief support groups will result in options within the area. There are also online groups and discussion boards available for advice and guidance. Many individuals who struggle with grief and require further support may benefit from psychology therapy or counseling. Many organizations offer this benefit and human resources may keep a list available for family and staff. Employee assistance programs may also be provided as an employee benefit and offer a set number of counseling sessions to staff. Finally, chaplain and spiritual support may offer family and staff comfort during difficult transitions in accepting and dealing with patient loss.

Organ Donation

Nurses should be aware of state and facility policies regarding organ donation. Rules and regulations differ according to state; however, the main role of the nurse is to facilitate the timely reporting of the death to the Organ Procurement Organization involved with screening for viability of organs and preparing the body until the organ harvesting team can retrieve it. Federal law mandates that any

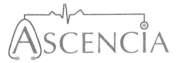

conversation surrounding organ donation is completed by a certified professional who represents an Organ Procurement Organization. When a patient has registered as an organ donor, this decision is considered to be legally binding. If the patient has not registered, the decision is made by the healthcare proxy or the next of kin.

There are certain criteria that typically exclude organ donation including diabetes, cancer, hepatitis, infectious disease, and organ disease; however, corneas may still be able to be donated.

Another significant role of the bedside nurse is to provide support and education to the family of the patient. This can involve allowing time with the patient to grieve prior to transporting for harvesting, explaining the process, and providing information about the effects that organ donation may have on individuals who are on the transplant waiting list.

Requirements for Reporting Death

When a patient dies, the nurse is responsible for simultaneous tasks that must be completed within a short time frame while still providing support to the family. Often the nurse will have other patients that still require care. Assessment of concurrent obligations and delegation of the care of other patients should be considered. The nurse should immediately notify the charge nurse for guidance and reassignment of other patients, if necessary.

When the nurse believes that death is impending, it is standard practice to notify the attending medical doctor. This courtesy gives the provider the opportunity to contact the family upon death. Depending on the state, the time of death can be pronounced by the medical doctor or by two nurses. If the provider is not available, the physician must be contacted as soon as possible after the nurse performs a final assessment. This assessment should be documented and include the date and time of the assessment, patient name, time that the physician was contacted, individuals present with the patient at the time of death, and the absence of apical pulse auscultation.

Upon patient death and notification to the physician and family, the nurse must determine if the coroner or medical examiner needs to be informed. This varies between states; however, there are generally defined circumstances where an autopsy will be performed, and facility policy should align with state requirements. These include death within 24 hours of admission to the hospital; the use of physical restraints; accidents, suicides, or homicides; drug intoxication or poisoning; sudden, unexpected, or suspicious deaths; deaths occurring outside of a medical care facility (with the exception of hospice cases); and deaths that are related to a medical or surgical procedure. The responsibility of notifying the coroner or medical examiner falls on the attending physician; however, the nurse should ensure that this has been completed and documented in the patient's chart.

The nurse may notify the family that the death has been reported to the medical examiner or coroner based on state guidelines. The decision to perform an autopsy on the patient will be determined following an investigation by the coroner's office and law enforcement.

Elements of Interprofessional Care

Nursing Process/Clinical Judgment Measurement Model

Nursing Process

The nursing process is a cyclical, systematic framework for patient assessment, diagnosis, planning, implementation, and evaluation. It is a fluid and dynamic methodology that ensures that patient care is approached in a standardized manner to collect data that can be analyzed to determine the patient's actual and potential care needs. Goals are set that align with the patient's identified diagnosis, and a plan is implemented that incorporates nursing interventions with physician orders for a comprehensive and holistic care plan. Once the intervention has been completed, the nurse uses critical thinking to evaluate the patient's response. The nursing process is effective because it allows forward movement or reversal based on the patient's individualized responses to evidence-based interventions.

The nursing process can be utilized as a tool that facilitates nursing care. Its most valuable characteristic is the ability to move through the components in a very fluid manner based on the patient's status. This includes moving forward and backward along the continuum or even reverting to the assessment based on the patient's presentation. Planning is reliant upon the assessment data identifying the immediate nursing diagnosis.

With the ever-changing patient condition, data may also change at any point during the nursing process, requiring a pivot from previous planning and goals. Utilizing the nursing process allows for quick adaptation and change to provide optimal focus on health delivery efforts that meet the patient's healthcare needs.

Assessment

A patient's health information is collected and documented through a holistic and comprehensive approach. Physiological, psychological, spiritual, economic, and other lifestyle factors that could be related to the patient's health are taken into account. The patient's history is obtained and reviewed for pertinence to current conditions and potential exacerbations. Any history within the medical record should be reviewed and verified with the patient. The patient's family members may be helpful if the patient is a poor historian. The physical assessment, also referred to as a head-to-toe assessment, provides valuable information to the nurse regarding the patient's disease process, progression, and manifestations of symptoms. Data may also come in the form of diagnostic tests such as X-rays, laboratory values, and ECGs.

The data that is gathered can be branched into two categories: subjective and objective. Subjective data is qualitative and based on the patient's perceptions, experiences, opinion, and feelings. Subjective data is more often used to describe symptoms such as dizziness, pain, feeling sick, or having an itch. This information is detailed by the patient verbally or in writing and provides the healthcare team with

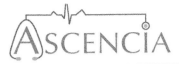

information about the patient's mindset about their symptoms and gravity of health concerns. It is important to explore this data, as it will shed light on what the patient feels are the most important parts of their healthcare. These may not align with the clinical concerns the healthcare team feels are most urgent to treat but may be more related to effects on the patient's daily activities and lifestyle.

Objective data is overt information that is conducive to signs of health. This information may be perceived, measured, and observed. The true test of whether data may be classified as objective is whether it can be verified and validated. This may be completed through observation using the senses, such as vision, smell, touch, or sound; via diagnostic procedures; or through laboratory studies.

A comprehensive assessment is a thorough and methodical gathering of the patient's medical and surgical history, body systems history and current functional status, current medication use, last time medications were taken, allergies, vital signs, and any patient safety requirements, such as assistive devices. This information is taken by the nurse and entered or updated in the patient's medical record.

A focused assessment is a condensed version of the former in that it specifically targets a particular disease process or system, such as cardiac or pulmonary. This is especially useful during critical or emergency situations when succinct information is needed quickly to make determinations on the patient's health status. Nurses must use critical thinking to ascertain the crucial details that need to be communicated to the healthcare team.

During an acute health episode, the nurse must triage a patient for symptoms. Strong clinical knowledge and critical thinking are needed to identify real or potential life-threatening emergencies. These characteristics are paramount to identifying the clinical information that is most concerning and related to the patient's immediate health emergency. Critical thinking may be described as a cognitive process combined with perception based on experience that may be applied to analyzing, synthesizing, and evaluating presented information to be quickly disseminated to drive interventions. This expertise is required during medical emergencies, especially those that may deviate from textbook descriptions. An example of this would be a female presenting with jaw pain and referred left shoulder pain. Since this is not the typical pain that would be associated with a myocardial infarction, critical thinking must be applied to recognize that females may have atypical symptoms such as jaw pain, back pain, or even just substernal indigestion feelings and should be worked up with a cardiovascular focused assessment.

Documentation should reflect the steps of the nursing process to effectively capture the data needed to contribute to the patient's care plan. Clear documentation of assessments will be an asset when comparing data once an intervention and reassessment has been completed. The record may be utilized to review attempted and successful outcomes. As this information is available to the multidisciplinary team, timely and comprehensive updates will keep the team updated on the patient's progress and any need for adjustments to the care plan.

Diagnosis

Nursing diagnoses are unique within the patient's healthcare plan. Unlike a medical diagnosis, which is a specific disease or condition, the nursing diagnosis is a judgment based on nursing knowledge to identify and understand the body system's response to a condition, process, or symptom. The nursing diagnosis describes the effects of the medical diagnosis; for example, a pulmonary embolism or pneumonia would have a nursing diagnosis of impaired gas exchange related to symptomatic presentation.

The nursing diagnosis is used to guide nursing interventions. These diagnoses are taken from a list of approved, standardized, and peer-reviewed recommendations for NANDA International (NANDA-I), which was formerly known as the North American Nursing Diagnosis Association. Per NANDA-I, the

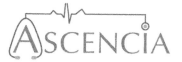

nursing diagnosis is "a clinical judgment concerning a human response to health conditions/life processes, or a vulnerability for that response, by an individual, family, group or community. A nursing diagnosis provides the basis for selection of nursing interventions to achieve outcomes for which the nurse has accountability" (Nanda International, 2023).

The medical diagnosis and data garnered from the assessment must be reviewed with an analytical mind, determining the most important information and what the true problem is that will provide the patient with the most efficacious outcomes. With this problem-focused approach, the signs, symptoms, and clinical presentation of the disease guide the nursing diagnosis selection. Similar to the previous example, a myocardial infarction that presents as chest pain, diaphoresis, pallor, and hypotension would lead to a nursing diagnosis of acute pain and risk for decreased cardiac output. Other nursing diagnoses would include fear/anxiety, risk for ineffective tissue perfusion, and activity intolerance. The nursing diagnosis is written systematically by stating the problem, relating it to the pathophysiology, and evidencing with the signs and symptoms presented. For pulmonary embolism, this may be written as: **Ineffective gas exchange** related to embolic obstruction as evidenced by ECG changes, tachycardia, shortness of breath, and feelings of impending doom.

From these nursing diagnoses, the nurse must triage what the focus will be when entering the planning stage of the nursing process. The goals that are identified and established within the planning phase must be derived from the nursing diagnosis, which makes this part of the process so essential to accurately identify the patient's priority clinical manifestations based on the medical diagnosis. Further, this accentuates the importance of a thorough assessment, which is relied upon by the interdisciplinary healthcare team to assist in formulating both the medical and nursing diagnosis.

Nanda International. (2023). Glossary of terms. In *Publications & Resources.* Retrieved from https://nanda.org/publications-resources/resources/glossary-of-terms/

Planning

Based on the priority needs identified from the assessment data and nursing diagnosis, the planning phase is the time during which the nurse plans care. Depending on the patient's health and comorbidities, many diagnoses may be identified. The nurse should use a prioritization framework, such as Maslow's hierarchy of needs, to translate the diagnosis to essential outcomes. The fundamental physiological needs must first be addressed. In healthcare, the priority is the ABCs: airway, breathing, and circulation. Short-term goals focus on returning the patient to a stable or baseline status. With medical emergencies, short-term goals may focus solely on returning spontaneous circulation after cardiopulmonary resuscitation or on improving oxygenation with mechanical ventilation.

Goals and outcomes are targeted at directly impacting the patient's care through the use of evidence-based guidelines. For the example of a pulmonary embolism, outcomes would focus on maintaining an open airway, promoting circulation, and anticipating diagnostic studies or treatments that would be applied to the disease process. For a pulmonary embolism, a goal may be to maintain adequate gas exchange, as evidenced by an oxygen saturation greater than 90% with the patient remaining fully alert and oriented.

For goals to be effective, they must follow a methodology that sets up success and achievability. A common format follows the acronym SMART (Specific, Measurable, Achievable, Relevant, and Time-based). A specific goal is a clearly defined and concise statement with one focal point. An example would be to maintain a patient's blood pressure within normal limits. Adding parameters to this goal would make it measurable. It is important to ensure that the parameters and measurements of the goal are

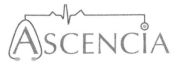

within reason and attainable. When reviewing the applicability of the outcome, it must align with the nursing diagnosis. Finally, the goal should have a specified time frame. For example, if blood pressure remains above a certain parameter at a certain point after treatment, the provider is notified. This ensures that the nursing process is being revisited and assessed frequently to provide the best outcomes possible.

As noted above, the nursing process is fluid, with capabilities to move from one phase to another and back again to ensure that the patient is continually assessed and that planning is revisited for optimal effects. The planning process may also be adjusted based on expertise, consultation, and feedback from other disciplines within the patient care team. Specialists within other branches of knowledge may offer insight to the planning process that is adjuvant to the patient's progress and goals. As the patient's condition changes, which can mean improvements or fallbacks, the planning process may require adjustments to meet the patient's needs. Planning will also change based on the patient's movement through the healthcare continuum.

Implementation

Implementation is the culmination of action via interventions from the planning phase. Interventions are treatments that are delivered to the patient based upon critical thinking, clinical judgment, knowledge, and education. These interventions may be nursing-derived or medically ordered within the plan of care. They include administering medications or oxygen, providing direct or indirect care, telemetry interpretation, and other therapeutic treatments. Implementations may be performed by the nurse or delegated, where appropriate. The nurse must follow up on any delegated intervention to ensure appropriate completion and that patient safety was maintained. Any intervention must be reassessed for patient response and effectiveness. Documentation in the medical record should include the date, time, nursing intervention completed, vital signs pre- and post-intervention, and whether the intervention produced the desired effects to meet the outcome. This information should be relayed to the healthcare team to update them and determine the next steps in the patient's care plan.

There are seven accepted nursing intervention domains. The physiological domain may be basic or complex. There are also behavioral, community, family, health system, and safety domains. Nursing interventions may be described by three categories: dependent, independent, and collaborative. Dependent nursing interventions are ones that must be ordered and delegated by an advanced care provider and within the nurse's area of expertise and knowledge. These interventions may not be initiated by the nurse alone. An example would be inserting an intravenous (IV) catheter. An independent nursing intervention would be one that is within the nurse's scope of practice, such as ambulating, repositioning, or obtaining vital signs from a patient. Collaborative nursing interventions are those that are team oriented. An example is a nurse collaborating with the physical therapist prior to a therapeutic exercise session to provide pain medication.

Evaluation

The last phase of the nursing process is evaluation. The subjective and objective data from the implementations are reassessed and compared against the goals to determine whether the goals were met, partially met, or not met within the parameters and time frames that were established during the planning phase. Each time an intervention is completed, this process must occur. It is a process that is continually performed depending upon the patient's condition. This guides the plan of care to either continue because the interventions have been successful or be revised. It falls just before assessment, as the interpretation of the evaluation leads to a new assessment of the patient's condition, signs, symptoms, or tolerance.

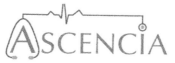

The evaluation phase is dependent upon the strength of the previously set goals and outcomes. This is why it is important to set goals that are SMART. Such goals will help the care team decide whether the intervention truly met the purpose of the treatment. For an intervention to be successful, the patient's condition should be improved to the parameters set forth in the planning stage and achieved within the time frame. The nurse must use critical thinking, observation, and communication skills. When the data is subjective, communication between the patient and the nurse is essential in determining whether the goals were met. This may include evaluating the pain level, shortness of breath, or itching. Both subjective and objective data must be accurately communicated to the healthcare team and documented in the electronic health record.

With this evaluation, the healthcare team must use the data, observations, and feedback from the patient to decide whether the implementation met the goals and whether the reassessment is satisfactory to meeting that patient's healthcare needs and agreed-upon outcomes. The care plan may be adjusted if the evaluation finds that some but not all outcomes were met. A medication or treatment may be added to the current regimen to increase the probability that the patient will respond effectively with additive or adjuvant care. If the evaluation finds that the patient is progressing within the time frame and parameters set in the planning phase, the treatment plan and interventions are continued. There are times when the evaluation shows that the patient is not responding well or cannot tolerate the treatment plan. In this case, the care plan is discontinued. This may also occur if the treatment was successful and is no longer needed. An example of this is a patient with a fluid volume deficit ordered to have a 1 L bolus of normal saline delivered via IV. If the patient responds to the treatment, their vital signs improve, and they return to baseline, the treatment is complete. Evaluation continues to be an evolving and continual process of reassessment and comparison against the other phases within the nursing process.

Interprofessional Collaboration

Role within the Interdisciplinary Team

Clear Team Member Roles

Role clarification must occur when the assigned care team is initially formed. This may change frequently while under the direction of the interdisciplinary team. Changes may occur during a single visit or shift or on a daily basis. A handoff report is a common method to establish accountability and responsibility among the team members. This defines the care that has occurred, interventions planned, and review tasks that are to be completed by each team member as well as who is being delegated responsibilities. There may be a conversation with the entire team, but typically, this report is done within the singular roles. The assigned nurse reports to the oncoming nurse prior to relinquishing care of the patient. Aides may also report to each other on the patient's activities of daily living, the mobility status of the patient, and any important events that occurred during that shift and then report to the nurse for further direction on the care plan for that shift.

This type of role clarification is also critical to establish during emergencies. For responders to a code situation, a primary lead should be quickly identified who then delegates roles to the other members of this team. Ensuring that all members have knowledge of their role prevents delays in care and confusion about expected interventions and encourages members to function as an effective team.

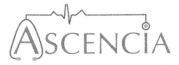

Communication Skills

While working within an interdisciplinary team, communication among all providers, nurses, unlicensed assistive personnel, and other disciplines involved in the care of the patient is a requirement to promote patient safety and integrate care that is comprehensive and patient centered. The healthcare environment is in constant momentum and may be chaotic. Ineffective or lost communication may result in patient harm because critical information is not received or is misinterpreted. Platforms that enhance communication are instituted within facilities to prevent these potential failures of information and facilitate the transmission of key updates by members of the healthcare team.

Policies will set rules for methods of communication for critical results, contacting providers, expectations of return communication, and updates for changes in patient status. Often, organizations will adopt electronic platforms and devices, such as a communication application that allows texting, video and phone calls, file and schedule sharing, and a real-time method to share and discuss patient care information. These tools allow the interdisciplinary healthcare team to quickly share and disseminate information when unable to engage in face-to-face conversation. Another common method of information sharing is using whiteboards in the patient's room to update the team on the patient's status, goals, mobility, and other key information needed to promote patient safety and keep care consistent and in line with the patient's care plan.

Interprofessional Rounding

For interdisciplinary bedside rounding to be effective, many disciplines involved in the care team should participate. This is not always feasible with the constraints of staffing, timing, and inability to coincide with other duties and responsibilities. At a minimum, however, it should include the nurse, the physician, and the patient. If possible, any specialty practices that are currently directing active care; placing orders and interventions; or overseeing planned or complete procedures, diagnostic tests, or surgeries should also attend.

If attendance is not possible, it is advisable that the disciplines that will be present at bedside report reach out to receive an update on any results, recommendations, or adjustments to the current care plan to enhance awareness for the entire care team and the patient. If the patient has further questions that cannot be addressed during the bedside report, the care team present may consult for further guidance or explanation and request further communication from the absent disciplines.

Formal interdisciplinary rounding is a planned event that typically involves addressing a broad topic rather than individual patient care. It may be referred to as a systems redesign project or root cause analysis and involve areas outside of clinical care, such as patient safety, leadership, and informatics. The topics that are focused on are usually qualitative and metrics driven. These may include reducing surgical turnover times or readmission rates or improving patient satisfaction scores. Data is gathered from clinical staff and patients through observation, surveillance, chart reviews, and audits. This data is disseminated and reviewed for trends, direct causes, and contributing factors so that action plans may be developed and implemented to improve the outcomes of the processes.

Care Coordination

Care for a patient often involves one or more disciplines working together. Team members should review the care plan and ensure that the interventions that are ordered and planned will align with the overall schedule of the interdisciplinary team. A strategy to keep all care providers on track is to hold care conferences. These may review several patients, either as a unit or within the team's responsibility,

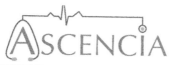

or discuss a single patient. During this time, disciplines may collaborate with each other to develop a plan that integrates care that should be aligned and timed appropriately.

Care team members may initiate conversations with other departments, such as rehabilitation, dietary, or social services, to facilitate care that will be optimal, convenient, or most beneficial to the patient. An example of this is for the dietary department to touch base with the nursing staff to discuss the delivery time of meal trays for patients who have diabetes. This allows the nurse to check the blood sugar and administer ordered insulin prior to the patient eating. Care planning and coordination deliberately establishes focused efforts to implement activities for optimal patient benefit.

Collaborative Problem Solving

Patient care is complicated, with multiple nuances that are managed by a team of disciplines including primary care providers, specialists, nursing, therapists, dieticians, and many others. All play equally important roles in managing the patient's health goals and work together to promote homeostasis to the patient's health. Disease treatment and symptom management is multifactorial, and the interdisciplinary team must work together to analyze the patient's condition, signs, and symptoms to critically evaluate the most effective means of promoting health and disease management.

Each member of the interdisciplinary team contributes expertise in their field of study. Collaboration to pool the knowledge from all disciplines must be established through respectful communication, openness to ideas, and information sharing. These tenets promote the professional integration of expert judgment within the changing dynamics of a patient's care continuum. The critical thinking process among the interdisciplinary team must be applied consistently, at regular intervals, and when the patient's clinical condition changes to drive cohesive, coordinated care.

Care Coordination and Transition Management

Interdisciplinary Collaboration Integration Methods

Discharge Planning

Safety is always the focus when the nurse is anticipating the needs of the patient post-hospitalization. In order to align care and bridge the gap between the patient's needs and resources to meet outcomes, the discharge planning process must start with admission. Once a patient is discharged, they are solely responsible for performing their daily activities, taking ordered medications as directed, following up with other care providers, and continuing treatments and outpatient care such as physical therapy.

The patient's educational, emotional, and physical ability to perform tasks and understand care moving beyond the hospital setting must be assessed as soon as possible to determine feasibility. The circle of support the patient has at home must be determined. It must not be assumed that the patient's family or other individuals will be amenable to caring for the patient outside the facility. When a caregiver who will be involved in the patient's care in the outpatient setting is identified, this support system must be established and involved in discussion with the interdisciplinary care team.

Each patient's care plan and discharge instructions should take into consideration the patient's lifestyle and culture and be patient-centered. A drive to ensure success for the patient outside the healthcare system is the push to reduce readmission rates. This is tied to certain financial incentives from reimbursement rates. Readmission of patients for the same diagnosis within a certain time frame may

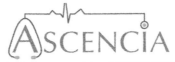

result in severe financial penalties. It is in the best interest of the patient and the organization to provide the patient with the coordination of care, resources, and follow-up care established prior to a transition of care to a rehabilitation facility or to home. Resources may come in the form of financial or other assistance from nonprofit or governmental sources and aim to ensure that the patient will be able to meet outcomes and maintain safety within the home. An example of aligning resources to ensure the patient's needs are met through the continuum of care is a patient who will require a wheelchair once discharged, with the nurse identifying through an assessment of the patient's home environment that there are stairs to enter the house. By identifying this need early, resources may be acquired that facilitate a handicap ramp being built to enter the patient's home. This type of collaboration takes time and involves multiple agencies and resources in order to be accomplished.

Communication within the interdisciplinary care team is essential to identify early barriers to discharge. The initial decision to discharge a patient will be made by the attending provider in concordance with specialties involved in the patient's care. This discharge plan will be discussed with the nurse and include the parameters the patient must meet to ensure safe discharge, a time frame, and the plan of care post-discharge. It is important that the nurse be diligent in assessing the patient's unique situation and informing the care team of any concerns the patient may have about managing care. An assessment should also include determining any equipment the patient may need and working with the department and insurance specialists that would assist in obtaining it for the patient prior to discharge (e.g., pharmacy to obtain a glucometer, testing strips, and lancets for a newly diagnosed diabetic). Early and frequent communication with the interdisciplinary care team is key to optimizing a successful patient discharge that promotes continued healing and ensures that safety is not compromised. Realization of these goals depends upon collaboration in decision-making through patient-centered care, interdisciplinary teamwork, agreeing upon goals set early on, and succinct, comprehensive education.

Barriers to Successful Care Coordination

Poor Interdisciplinary Teamwork and Communication

Patient safety is intrinsically linked to accurate and effective communication within the interdisciplinary healthcare team. Poor communication can lead to misunderstanding of information conveyed, misinterpreting orders, unrecognized clinical status changes, and missing critical information.

An organization, whether it is a small agency or a large facility, must promote collaboration, trust, and respect, the key elements of effective communication. This can be done by applying policies and procedures to apply expectations from the top down. Promoting executive leadership rounding to address concerns and inform staff breaks one of the most common struggles with interpersonal power and conflict—hierarchical differences. Promoting a "see something, say something" culture is also an effective way to encourage acceptance of open conversation and reduce the negative impact that poor communication can have on patient care.

With a rising population and an increase in lifespan, chronic disease and higher acuity levels have led to increased stress, difficulty meeting role expectations, and lower performance. Burnout due to increased nurse-to-patient ratios increases the likelihood of lack of engagement. With seemingly not enough time to perform all duties, staff may opt to attempt to curtail standards of care and cut back on performing all steps that are normal for a procedure. Partial or complete omission of patient care or communication with the interdisciplinary team puts patients at risk. These violations have high implications for decreasing quality and safety.

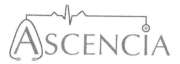
Since "meaningful use" of electronic health records became federally mandated, there has been an uptick in different types of digital medical and health records. This initiative and law was intended to improve quality and safety, engage patients and family with expanded access to their health records, and improve care coordination. Unfortunately, with the vast array of records, there is difficulty in obtaining information across different systems. There may be multiple digital records used across one organization, dependent upon the type of department and its use of them. Rather than the initial vision of having open and flowing communication that is quick and efficient, if systems do not align, the process for obtaining records is slow and requires verification of need and use of older methods of transmission, such as mail, fax, or email. The ramifications of this are delays in care, fragmented information, missing records, and inaccurate or outdated data that leads to compromised patient care.

Discharge Procedures

Medication Reconciliation

Medication reconciliation is a process that reviews each medication that a patient is taking and compares that to all medications that are currently ordered. Each medication is verified and validated with the patient against the medical record for name, dose, timing, and reason for treatment. At each transition of care, medication reconciliation should be completed to prevent medication errors, including dosing errors, drug interactions, omissions, and duplications. There are five steps to completing the medication reconciliation process. First, a current medication list must be entered into the medical administration record. This is obtained from the patient or caregiver during the admission assessment. When the patient is not able to provide this information, the pharmacy that the patient has used may be contacted for an up-to-date list. Second, the admitting provider must review these medications and determine which medications will continue as well as input any new medications that have been ordered and administered with the current treatment plan. Third, these lists must be compared. Fourth, clinical decisions must be made based on the comparison. At this time, any nonactive medications will be discontinued, and any medications to continue will be added to the current medication administration record. Finally, these changes are communicated to the care team. When new orders are received, the nurse must verify and note them within the electronic health record.

Records and Discharge Paperwork

During the discharge process, the medications will again be reviewed and compared against the patient's original medication record. All medications previously taken in the outpatient setting will be assessed for continuation, safety, and any contraindications with new medications. The new list will be updated with all medications that will be continued post-hospitalization as well as medications that should be discontinued. The nurse will review these thoroughly with the patient and assess understanding with teach-back and knowledge checks. A list of all new medications, dosages, timing, and time last taken will be provided to the patient. The medications that are to be discontinued should also be clearly stated within the discharge instructions.

Most medical records include the functionality of a disease process library that covers pathophysiology, common treatments, complications, and when to seek medical attention. This type of education should be tailored to the patient's condition, learning preferences, and knowledge level. Paperwork for discharge will also include the reason for the patient's admission, the updated medication list, upcoming appointments, any scheduled procedures and surgeries, and signs and symptoms to be aware of. The nurse completing the discharge will review the entirety of the discharge papers with the patient, assess

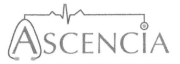

understanding, and facilitate individual provider or interdisciplinary team discussion if the patient requires further information.

Care Coordination

Care management should continue throughout the entirety of the discharge process, starting from admission. Keeping all members of the interdisciplinary team informed provides solidarity on the treatment plan. Each member of the team should be cognizant of their own specialty's projected care, including awaiting diagnostic tests to guide further treatment, any upcoming procedures, and other timely matters that may affect the planning that will go into the patient's discharge. Coordinating care to be aligned with an agreed-upon timeline will provide the interdisciplinary team with a framework for planning care. Interdisciplinary rounds should continue until discharge. During this time, the care team can coordinate and communicate the care that will be provided in the outpatient setting and review expectations of wellness and outcomes in the transition of care.

Patient/Family Centered Care

Throughout the patient's admission to a healthcare facility, the healthcare team will coordinate education related to any treatment, intervention, or new equipment or device that will need to be managed post-hospitalization. Education and teaching should begin as soon as the patient and care team have elected to perform the medical intervention. The nurse should initially establish the learner's preferred style. Education may begin with introducing the new treatment via demonstration, literature, or an informational video. Throughout the hospital stay, the nurse may include the patient and/or caregiver in the process.

An example of this would be for a patient who has received a tracheostomy tube. The above-referenced teaching may begin at the bedside during the preparation phase and be incorporated into the informed consent process. Once the procedure is complete, the nurse may involve the patient and caregiver in incisional care; review precautions while healing occurs; and demonstrate suctioning of the tube, tube changes, infection prevention, and how to manage mucus plugs. As the patient approaches the time to discharge, the patient and family should be incrementally more hands-on with the care, with the goal that the patient and caregiver feel comfortable managing the ostium and ensuring that the tube stays patent.

The patient-centered care model focuses on aligning care with the patient's preferences, needs, and values. The healthcare team must consider the patient beyond their disease process and the immediate events. To achieve success with patient compliance and outcomes within the continuum of care, the patient's whole environment, ideals, socioeconomic status, available resources, and culture must be incorporated into the care plan. This requires developing a relationship with the patient that is guided by communication, trust, respect, and a commitment to accommodating perceived constraints and individually challenging circumstances.

Between the expansion of the internet and commitments by communities to improve their populations' health, many patient resources are readily available. The nurse should be educated and adept at locating and connecting system and community resources to coordinate patient care. These resources may include support groups, educational sessions, assistance for disadvantaged groups, and other social services. Often, a facility or nursing unit will keep a list of various resources to connect the patient to prior to discharge.

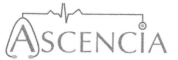

Care Coordination and Transition

Creating a clear patient portrayal through health assessments has multiple facets from many different sources. Previous encounters through the healthcare system provide a clinical perspective and establish previous, current, and planned treatment. The medical record is a valuable resource for maintaining the history of the patient and should include information from multiple sources. Nursing and clinical notes are often first referred to for gathering data about a patient. Other sources may include respiratory therapy, dietary, and physical therapy notes. Mental health and clergy may also provide information that can enhance the understanding of the patient through different perspectives.

First and foremost, information should come from the patient. Conducting a detailed interview and assessment of the patient in addition to reviewing the chart will augment any data that is revealed. A patient's family or friends, with the patient's permission, may also be valuable players in providing a clearer understanding of the patient's health, habits, lifestyle, and adherence to medical compliance, along with general knowledge of the patient.

A patient will go through multiple transitions of care and movement through different settings, including changes in care providers during shift changes, movement with escalation or de-escalation of care, and interfacility transfers. Whenever a patient's care team changes, a report must be delivered that covers at a minimum the patient's history, current clinical assessment, medications, concerns, and a review of provided and upcoming patient care. The Joint Commission recommends that the process of a handoff report is standardized and is acknowledged as a transfer of responsibility for patient care. This measure promotes patient safety, keeps team members updated, and enhances communication. Transitions to different levels of care that are within the same facility may need to include additional information besides a shift report. This may include the patient's original diagnosis, the reason for the change in care, and certain documents from the medical record, such as a face sheet. Transfers that require ambulance transport will also require a report to the emergency medical services team that will assume care during transportation. To promote standardization, a form with the key, required patient information that is communicated during the verbal report is recommended. This will be sent with the patient to the accepting facility and staff for review. Callback numbers for the previous facility and caregiver are included in case clarification or a review of any information is needed.

To assist patients in being adequately connected with referrals, the nurse should ensure that the referrals are ordered and that the service line is notified of the patient's transition. If possible, the discharging nurse may reach out to the service to schedule the initial appointment. The time and date of the appointment may then be included with the discharge instructions to provide a reference for upcoming care.

The patient and family and/or the facility that the patient is being transferred to, if applicable, must be updated with the name and contact information of the company providing services, how often the therapy or treatment should occur, and the dates and times of scheduled appointments.

Continuum of Care

A patient's care may follow many different pathways. Care may be first established in a preventive care setting, such as a primary care office. The patient's conditions may be identified, monitored, and managed with medical treatment. At times, a patient may only see healthcare providers intermittently or on an as-needed basis. An emergency department visit due to a medical incident may initiate introduction to the medical care system. Each patient will have a slightly different pathway into the continuum of care. This continuum will provide the care that patients require at each stage.

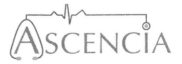

When a patient has an event that requires emergent care, the patient will be triaged within the emergency department to determine the severity of illness or injury, with the main goal being stabilization. It will be determined whether the patient requires an escalation of care depending on the scope of their symptoms. In some cases, the patient may be stabilized at that point with treatment and released to home with a plan to follow up with a primary care provider or specialist. If the patient's clinical condition is severe or may require several days of treatment, the patient will be admitted to the facility. There are levels of care within nursing units in the hospital, including medical-surgical, oncological, progressive, cardiovascular, and critical care, to tend to a patient's unique conditions.

Once the patient is stabilized and deemed medically appropriate to discharge from the hospital setting, the interdisciplinary care team must decide on the best route for the patient to continue receiving care in order to return to baseline. The patient may return home with little to no further need for care. If the patient requires assistance with activities of daily life, depending on the support the patient may already have within the home, a home care agency may provide skilled nursing care to bridge the gap. Outpatient rehabilitation, which may include occupational, speech, or physical therapy, can be arranged as needed.

There are instances where returning home directly post-hospitalization would not be conducive to the patient's healing process or health goals. In this case, a subacute rehabilitation facility or skilled nursing care facility would provide the patient with increased assistance, especially in cases where mobility or safety is a concern.

During this journey, a patient may be seen by multiple providers, specialists, and care teams. Coordinating care is complex and challenging. Care provided by a healthcare organization is often not coordinated in a simplified and linear pattern, leaving the patient and family to manage appointments, scheduling of care, and regular communication with the agencies that are involved in the patient's care plan. Advocating for improved communication and information sharing among the interdisciplinary teams, specialists, and patient and family can facilitate the continuum of care to improve efficiency and decrease gaps of care. Nursing should be actively involved at all points along this timeline to provide education and resources to assist the patient with access to care as they move through this system.

Patients at Risk for Readmission

Readmission post-discharge is a possibility for many high-risk patients and has a higher occurrence with multiple chronic and acute comorbidities. A readmission is defined as a subsequent admission to an inpatient status within 30 days of being discharged for the same diagnosis. Factors that may increase the likelihood of readmission that may be preventable with interdisciplinary planning and coordination include inadequate post-discharge planning and support, lack of or delay in follow-up care, errors in therapy or medication, poor handoff reports, complications due to procedures, and early discharge.

There are also unmodifiable factors related to readmission. These include prior hospitalization within the past 6 to 12 months, having more than six chronic diagnoses, and the use of certain medications or polypharmacy. There are certain clinical conditions that are linked to readmission occurring. Patients afflicted with diabetes, heart disease, cerebrovascular accident, cancer, depression, sepsis, and respiratory conditions such as chronic obstructive pulmonary disorder have a higher rate of readmission than those with other diagnoses.

Certain nonclinical or non-disease-related conditions may also be more apt to readmission. Socioeconomic status and demographics can be linked to concurrent hospitalizations. Individuals with lower socioeconomic status, low health literacy, or lack of a social network and those who choose to

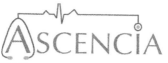

leave treatment against medical advice are more likely to return with exacerbation of the same disease process within 30 days.

According to statistics published by the Agency for Healthcare Research and Quality, close to 20 percent of patients experience a clinically significant adverse event within 3 weeks of being discharged. Of those events, around 75 percent may have been prevented or lessened in severity. The majority of adverse events are related to medication incidents. Readmission rates are directly tied to poor patient outcomes and higher mortality rates.

Healthcare facilities are graded on readmission rate metrics. Allowing rates to remain high affects reimbursement due to penalties incurred from Medicare. Publicly reported scores are unfavorable if readmission rates are higher than those of competing local organizations. Other significant effects include a higher overall cost of care, negative feedback and perceptions among the community, and lack of employee engagement.

Social Determinants of Health

Social determinants of health can have significant effects on health statistics and risk for poor outcomes. Being knowledgeable on the data within the local area can help mitigate risk and anticipate the health needs of the local population. It enables nurses and healthcare providers to aim efforts at preventive factors for the highest-risk health populations (e.g., individuals with diabetes), improve health outcomes, increase patient engagement, decrease rates of readmission, lower health organizational costs, and improve compliance with quality standards.

Individuals who reside in rural locations, have a low socioeconomic status, or identify within vulnerable populations are at an increased risk of experiencing difficulties obtaining healthcare, connecting with needed resources, and meeting health outcomes. Limited resources lead to difficulty obtaining or keeping health insurance, gaining access to a regular healthcare provider, and being able to afford prescription medications and regular healthcare treatment.

According to national public health publications, the major factors that affect health outcomes include employment, poverty, and education. These social determinants of health can also affect the ability to obtain safe and adequate housing, healthy foods, transportation, and media and technology.

Health literacy is the ability to obtain, understand, and decipher basic health information and to apply that to the decision-making process regarding effective, beneficial healthcare. Individuals with low health literacy are more likely to have frequent hospitalizations, use emergency care more often, lack access to preventive services, and have poor health outcomes. Mortality rates and healthcare costs are significantly higher in this population than in those with moderate to high healthcare literacy.

When individuals with low health literacy do seek treatment, they are more likely to seek medical attention when illness is advanced, leading to a delayed diagnosis. Outcomes are also likely to be less optimal due to a higher likelihood of a poorly managed disease and lack of compliance for weight management, tobacco usage, and recommended cancer screenings.

Individuals who have a higher risk for poor health literacy include those in the nonwhite population and those with low socioeconomic status, lack of higher-level education, and lower income. Individuals over 60 years of age and those whose native language is not English are also at an increased risk for having low health literacy.

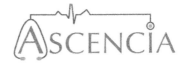

Quality Patient Outcome Measures

Quality measures are used to define an organization's overall wellness in comparison to other facilities of the same size and the same location. This is tracked by accreditation and national standards of care to guide organizational change and provide statistics for public knowledge. There are three categories of quality measures: structural, process, and outcome.

Structural measures include an organization's systems, processes, and ability to provide high-quality care. Measures included are related to patient-to-provider ratios, how many providers within the facility are board certified, and whether an electronic medical record and medication administration record are utilized.

Process measures involve the methods that are employed to maintain or improve health, for both preventive and maintenance care. These include the number of preventive services offered, such as immunizations and mammograms, as well as the number of individuals with diabetes who have their blood sugar tracked and controlled.

Outcome measures reveal the outcomes of interventions or services provided up to the overall health status of patients. Metrics include mortality rates with surgical procedures, rates of hospital-acquired infections, and other surgical complications.

Outcome measures are tracked by facilities to measure their own organizational health. Certain reporting is required for organizations participating in Medicaid and Medicare programs. There are core sets of measures and surveys, including the Consumer Assessment of Healthcare Providers and Systems survey, as well as certain measure sets for managed care. Other methods of obtaining data include standardized clinical data, comments from patients, targeted patient surveys, and auditing of medical records.

Documentation

Documentation of Patient Care

The purpose of the nursing record is to communicate and share pertinent, accurate, and meaningful information with healthcare providers and other individuals who are essential to the care of the patient. The nursing care plan, patient clinical and safety events, nursing care activities, results of tests, and progress notes are made available to a multi-disciplinary care team for review. Nursing documentation must capture accurate clinical data for the patient record to support safe, patient-centered care. All roles within the nursing discipline are charged with ensuring that documentation is legible, understandable, and correctly reflects the patient's presentation.

To capture an accurate record of the patient's chronological events, documentation should ideally be completed in real-time. If this is not possible, the nurse should backtime the data entered into the medical record to reflect the hour and minute that the event or care was provided. This will ensure that there is a verifiable depiction of events that can be sequentially followed. All documentation entered should be verified against clinically confirmed patient data. Providers rely upon this information to adjust the patient's plan of care. This is especially true with diagnostic tests, medication administration, and treatment adjustments that are dependent upon the patient's response. Vital signs, mental status, hemodynamic stability, or pulmonary status—along with other clinical signs and symptoms—must be

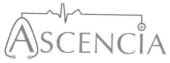

accounted for and accurately represented to safely proceed with treatment plans. This critical data should be entered into the medical record in real-time or as close to it as possible.

Without accurate documentation, the client's status is not reflected in a manner that provides information that can be appropriately utilized for treatment. Nurses must be aware and diligent to ensure that the documentation entered is correct. The nurse may oversee ancillary staff that may enter documentation, and the nurse is responsible for the verification of results or assessments entered. Documentation is relied upon to support meeting regulatory standards of care and to track key metrics that may be used for coding and billing. Unless the documentation can support the patient's diagnosis, support meaningful use, and confirm value-based care, insurance reimbursement may be withheld or denied. The documentation must portray a comprehensive and clear picture of the care provided to the patient.

The medical record is accessed for a variety of purposes and utilized by individuals with a myriad of backgrounds, education, and intentions for information use. Most commonly, the record is accessed by nurses and providers to update or be updated on the patient's condition and progress of care. Reasonable access to healthcare records is provided to patients. Family and caregivers authorized by the patient may be given access to a patient portal via an online platform. Patients may also request physical records of their healthcare. This is typically completed through the medical records department of the facility where care was received and may take several weeks to process. This information should be relayed to patients requesting access to their healthcare records. Nurses must never provide printouts or copies of the medical record directly to the patient.

Care should be taken to ensure that the data and narrative are clear, concise, and easy to read. It is important that the electronic health record displays content legibly on multiple platforms as it may be brought up on different electronic devices such as laptops, desktop computers, and cell phones.

Standardization supports consistency in care and provides for patient safety through adopting practices and standards that are evidence-based. Only universally approved acronyms should be utilized to avoid confusion and potential safety incidents. Each organization will have a specific standardized or approved list of acronyms that the nurse should become familiar with as well. Nursing documentation should be succinct, objective, and unbiased. There are several nursing documentation frameworks that may be used by healthcare entities to support standardization. These include charting by exception, narrative form, problem-focused charting, and systems-based documentation. Nursing representation is essential in choosing the style of standardization and promoting the singular use of the framework to avoid variation.

Nurses are not the sole authors of the medical record. Healthcare providers, respiratory therapists, physical therapists, dietary staff, chaplains, and any other individual employed or contracted by the healthcare organization may contribute to the patient record. These individuals must be included in the appropriate training for accessing, documenting, and upkeeping the patient record.

Documentation Platforms

Electronic health records (EHRs) are an accessible, multi-platform version of the patient's record that is in a digital format. These records contain information including demographics, diagnoses, healthcare history, past and present medications, allergen information, previous immunizations, laboratory data, vital signs, and results of diagnostic tests. Automated information is used to guide patient care by mapping trends and monitoring changes in results.

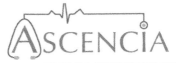

There are numerous electronic health records available on the market and most provide unique, customizable features based on the provider's or facility's needs. Some of the features that can enhance a clinical user's experience include decision support tools, embedded references (e.g., drug encyclopedias), alerts to critical values, and communication tools between providers and clinical staff.

EHRs were promoted as a key initiative in the drive for meaningful use in the United States. These are the standards set by the government to define how clinical data is shared between all parties relevant to the patient's record. This includes patients, healthcare providers, and insurers.

Research and evidence-based practice have shown that automatic and broad accessibility to patient records by appropriate providers and facilities increases patient safety through the reduction of medical errors.

Even during times when the electronic health record is not accessible, the nurse must ensure that patient documentation captures the correct clinical sequence of events. These events are typically referred to as "downtime" and may be planned or unplanned. Examples of planned downtime include system updates, equipment changes, other maintenance activities, and mock drills. An alert several days ahead of the scheduled downtime should be distributed to the users it will affect so that accommodations can be made. Natural disasters, internet or intranet disruptions, and equipment failure may also cause unplanned downtimes.

Both types of downtimes must be planned for in advance. Nurses are responsible for knowing the downtime procedures and policies of their workplace. Education on completing paper charting forms prior to downtime is important to establish expectations of documentation. These forms should be kept in a readily accessible location for ease of obtaining when needed. Updated patient demographics (sometimes called a "face sheet") and medication administration records will need to be printed and kept up to date in preparation for both planned and unplanned downtimes.

Performance Improvement in Documentation

Performance improvement projects aim to discover means of increasing proficiency, standardizing processes, and meeting goals that are quantifiable and agreed-upon objectives that align with the organization's standards. There are substantial opportunities for continuous improvement in the design, interface, and use of the electronic health record that aim to provide a user experience that enhances communication, speeds the flow of patient information delivery, reduces duplicity of orders, and enhances claim capture.

Projects are typically led by a team within information technology, with representation by nurse informaticists who focus on improving ease of use, patient safety checks and alerts, and capturing the data that nurses are involved in entering and verifying. They are responsible for working with leadership to develop documentation guidelines, procedures, policies, protocols, and standards.

Patient documentation that is poorly captured in the medical record or is not easily found or accessible may lead to poor patient outcomes. This is true across all clinical and outpatient settings. Interventions should be aimed at the goal, based on the setting, and be customizable and related to the data that is most pertinent to the patient's care. The nurse informaticists must be able to identify barriers to charting and impedances to the workflow that are experienced by the users.

An example of this may be in the documentation and follow-up for a pain assessment. To understand the process, the nurse informaticist must first analyze the function of the electronic health record to document this information. Then a determination may be made of modifications that would ease the

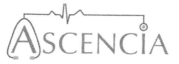

capture of the initial assessment as well as prompts to assist with the follow-up of any interventions. Other methods to create a safer patient experience may include reducing the number of clicks, creating shortcuts to commonly used data entry points, incorporating hard stops to alert providers, and inserting visual cues to prompt an action.

Technology

Equipment Use and Troubleshooting

IV Pump

Intravenous pumps, also referred to as external infusion pumps, are used to deliver intravenous solutions in a controlled, exact method via an electric or mechanical device. Precise flow rates are regulated via stepper or DC motors. Pre-loaded drug formularies are programmed into the smart pumps to provide a safeguard for upper and lower limits to medications and alert when these are triggered. Nurses are responsible for making sure that the correct dosages are calculated and entered based on orders, body weight, and other patient-specific factors.

Manufacturer's instructions on use and cleaning should be reviewed prior to use along with becoming familiar with the various alarms and their meanings. Settings are available to adjust for sound, digital screen brightness, and lock-out options.

When alarms sound, the cause should be investigated with the pump paused. One of the most common causes of alarms is low battery. Ensure that the IV pump is plugged in and charging. Another common cause for alarms is an impedance of flow, such as a kink in the IV tubing or a bend in the patient's arm. When priming the IV tubing, any bubbles should be allowed to flow through to prevent this from occurring.

If a pump is malfunctioning or not turning on, the medical device should be removed from service and submitted for repair to the biomedical department according to facility policy.

Bedside ECG Monitor

Bedside ECG monitoring is common in progressive, cardiac, and critical care units to monitor and record the cardiac electrical signal for dysrhythmias. Electrodes with conductive gel are placed at certain points on the chest. The electrodes are connected to the bedside monitor via clips or snaps.

Ensure that ECG patches are placed per order or facility policy in the appropriate location for the most accurate readings. Inaccurate readings may occur due to limited contact with the skin, movement, and inappropriate placement of electrodes. The skin should be dry, free of hair, and free of any oils or lotions.

Interference in the recordings may be due to any of these factors. It is important to verify dysrhythmias that appear on the monitor by assessing the patient prior to any treatment.

Feeding Tube Pump

Feeding tube pumps deliver enteral nutrition via a tube inserted through the nasogastric/orogastric path or via a stoma with a tube to the gastrointestinal system. In a similar way to the IV pump, this medical device provides automatic delivery of a nutritional formula through a feeding tube set. The set may

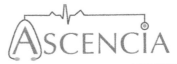

create an alarm due to a stop of flow. This may occur due to a blockage or kink in the line. It is important to thoroughly flush and change out the system per the manufacturer's guidelines.

Due to the high risk of aspiration, the system should be stopped for any alarms and the cause investigated. A chest x-ray to verify placement is the gold standard upon initiating any treatment. Placement should be verified prior to each use via pH testing of aspirated fluid or auscultation of an air bolus per facility policy.

Mechanical Ventilator

Mechanical ventilators may be set up and maintained by nursing or respiratory therapists depending on facility and state guidelines. When alarms sound on the ventilator, first ensure that the patient's oxygenation level is appropriate and that the patient is not in acute respiratory distress. If the patient is unstable, the ventilator should be disconnected, and the patient bag ventilated with 100 percent oxygen until assistance arrives.

Alarms may be due to high pressure or low pressure. High-pressure alarms are associated with a blockage and may be due to pulmonary edema, atelectasis, mainstem intubation, tension pneumothorax, pleural effusions, or consolidation. Low-pressure alarms are more consistent with a disconnected tube or lost airway. Placement of the endotracheal tube or tracheostomy tube should be verified as well as checking that the tubing joints are all appropriately connected along the system and that the connection to the machine is secure.

Technology Trends in Healthcare

The medical field is ever expanding to incorporate new technologies that improve patient care, safety, and accessibility. Telehealth, also referred to as virtual care, is a relatively new concept that brings the provider into the patient's home at their convenience. This was bolstered by the Covid-19 public health emergency, enabling appropriate and safe care to occur despite being in a remote location. The patient may participate in a clinical visit via telephone or video. This may be applied to multiple health services including clinical visits, counseling, physical and occupational therapy, home health, and management of chronic disease.

Artificial intelligence is being expanded and used more within the medical field as a tool to improve patient treatment. It is currently being used to increase the rate of malignant tumors being identified in radiological exams and improve the identification of arrhythmias and dysrhythmias in ECGs. Machine-based algorithms are being applied to earlier diagnostics of a multitude of diseases, standardization of analyzing medical data, and increasing access for vulnerable populations.

Since the 1980s, robotics have been increasingly used in surgical areas with the emergence of robotic arm technologies. These devices assist the surgeon with precision to reduce infections and speed healing in abdominal and orthopedic surgeries. The use of robotics has expanded since that time to modular robots that enhance rehabilitation and exercise, autonomous mobile robots that can provide wayfinding and supply delivery, and service robots that are capable of restocking, tracking supplies, and cleaning and sanitizing clinical areas.

Nursing Informatics

Nursing informatics is the science and practice of nursing information and knowledge. It is the basis of providing patient care by managing communication and information technologies to be fully integrated into the multidisciplinary team. The nursing informaticist plays an integral role within the information

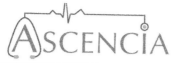

technology department. This role is the lifeline between the informatics department and the nursing body. By monitoring trends and data, the nursing informaticist can help identify areas to improve the technological processes that are used by nurses in the clinical setting. Barriers to charting, patient care, communication, and meeting charting guidelines are identified by the nursing informaticist and communicated with the IT team to develop solutions.

The nursing informaticist's role covers a broad range beyond representing clinical nursing within the IT department. This role expands from the bedside to policy development at a national level. While providing representation at all levels, the standards and processes that are advocated for should always be supported by evidence-based practice and upheld to the highest research and scholarly rigors. This research must be translated into working knowledge to improve practice and patient safety. Educating nursing staff and providers is a significant facet of the nursing informaticist's role. Also, the nurse informaticist must be able to provide a vision and plan to executive leadership that will guide patient workflow needs with a multidisciplinary focus.

Professional Concepts

Communication

Chain of Command

The chain of command is the administrative process followed to voice concerns and advocate on the patient's behalf when other interventions have not been successful. It is the duty of each nurse to be aware of the appropriate chain of command to escalate concerns. Each facility may have a slightly different organizational chart to follow; however, the process is similar. Every organization should have a policy developed that clearly delineates the purpose of escalating a concern and initiating the chain of command. Common reasons for these include the following: seeking guidance when concerns have not been addressed, clarifying a patient care plan, obtaining assistance to manage a care intervention, mitigating liability in support of risk management, and ensuring that the minimum standard of care is upheld and followed. These situations are especially true when differing opinions arise between the multidisciplinary team.

Many times, concerns for the patient are related to situations that may cause harm to the patient. The type and severity of harm are important to keep in mind when escalating these concerns and deciding how far up the chain to address concerns based on the responses of the previous administrative officer.

There are trends among concerns for patients that are consistently voiced. One of the most reported patient safety concerns is ambiguous patient orders, which may include medications or interventions. This may be due to illegibility, incompleteness, or contraindications with the patient's diagnosis or treatment plan. A patient's decline or worsening of symptoms that the nurse believes is not being addressed according to the minimum standard of care can also be a valid reason for initiating the chain of command.

At times there may be conflict between the patient and provider or clinical staff that is due to a disagreement on the patient's current treatment plan or care provided. Advance directives are important to address with each patient at the time of admission. When this is not accomplished or the expectations are not clearly established, there can be conflict due to ambiguity. This may occur when the patient becomes incapacitated and unable to make their own decisions, leaving the burden upon the next-of-kin or family to decide, leading to a potential for disagreement.

Most facilities have a set policy for provider response times. When this is not met, the nurse may need to escalate the requirement of the provider or a proxy to address concerns in a timely manner.

Nursing leadership is built upon a hierarchical chain. The clinical RN is responsible for tasks delegated to licensed professional nurses and nursing assistants. These assistive personnel should initially bring any patient safety concerns to the RN. The RNs on a unit are usually overseen each shift by a charge RN. This role may be a dedicated position or shared among the regular staff for each shift. Concerns should first be escalated from the assistive personnel staff or RN to the charge nurse. Depending on the shift, the chain of command then moves to either the unit manager or the hospital supervisor. The hospital supervisor is more readily available during off-hours, such as night shifts or weekends. If the concern still

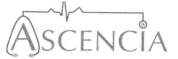

needs to be brought to an upper executive level, the chief nursing officer is the head of the nursing body. It is the responsibility of each part of the chain of command to investigate the situation and provide a plan of action.

The nurse that is escalating the concern must document the concerns, who they were reported to and the response, as well as any interventions provided related to this guidance. The chart should clearly provide a picture of the safety concern and follow through the course of action that was determined by the chain of command.

Communication Skills

Active Listening

Paramount to the success of providing care, education, and support to patients is the practice of effective communication. Active listening involves receiving the message, interpreting the meaning, and appropriately responding based on the speaker's needs. Using active listening techniques—such as attentiveness—while communicating with patients relieves anxiety by allowing the speaker time to share their perspective. Trust is earned as patients will feel they are being respected and their concerns are being taken seriously.

There are several other techniques that may be used to improve active listening. The nurse may repeat back to the patient what was understood to clarify the message and to increase attentiveness. This is known as paraphrasing and summarizing. Reflection may be used to understand feelings. Always phrase questions as open-ended to avoid leading and to gain more information.

Ensuring that the setting is appropriate with few distractions can also enhance active listening. This includes creating a private, safe environment in which the patient will feel secure in sharing private information. Any physical barriers, such as screens or obstructions that block anyone's view, should be removed, and the space should be free from external noise or distraction. Technology can also increase distractions. Any computers, telephones, or other technological devices should be silenced or, at least, on a low volume.

Proficiency in Communication Mediums

Communication is extremely important to the efficacy and functioning of the interdisciplinary team to meaningfully connect with patients. Building strong communication skills will enable nurses to adapt to different styles and educational levels and promote patient safety. Team members who are able to interact with each other and the patient contribute to optimizing patient outcomes and improving collaboration.

Verbal communication that is succinct, truthful, and clearly delivered prevents misunderstandings among the team members. The speaker should speak slowly, clearly, and use correct grammar. It is best to avoid slang terms as these may be interpreted differently based on education level, cultural factors, age, and region. These factors, along with any biases or presumptions that may be present, should be taken into consideration prior to the conversation occurring.

Body language and gestures may improve the perception of active listening. Using appropriate eye contact and open posture can help convey interest through positive body language. Personal space must be respected; however, it is important to ensure that conversations, especially regarding patient information, are not easily heard by other parties.

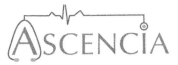

In healthcare, there is a wide variety of written communication to a vast audience including providers, patients, nursing, ancillary staff, leadership, and administrative personnel. Common communication mediums include but are not limited to memos, educational content, texts, website content, and patient records. Written communication should focus on being legible and professional with correct spelling and grammar. Follow facility policy for letterhead and formatting rules. It is important to keep education and communication with patients at a level easily understood by the majority of the population. Content should be created at a sixth to eighth grade reading level, according to the American Medical Association.

Empathy

Empathy is the state of expressing understanding and sharing another's feelings. This is different from sympathy where the feeling is of sorrow for another's misfortunes. Having the ability to share another's experience from a viewpoint where one can understand the situation, their reactions, and the gravity of their emotions and feelings allows one to comprehend from a unique perspective. This is helpful in allowing patients to express themselves without fear of shame, bias, or judgment.

Psychologists promote three types of empathy: emotional, cognitive, and compassionate. Emotional empathy is when the listener can experience the same emotions as the speaker. This helps to build a deeper connection between individuals and can be used as a technique to develop an understanding of the behaviors of patients. Cognitive empathy creates an understanding of the speaker's perspective from a logical viewpoint. This is useful during high-stress situations and when there are multiple factors or frames of reference. Finally, compassionate empathy is an understanding of the speaker's concern and the desire to assist to alleviate the matter.

Empathy is an important tool for communication as it promotes an open attitude towards understanding and embracing another's experiences and feelings without bias or condemnation. This supports the concept of patient-centered care by allowing the patient to share in a mind-frame that is conducive to acceptance.

Conflict Resolution and Mediation

The healthcare environment can be stressful, and conflict may arise between any members of the healthcare team. Healthy responses to conflict can improve relationships, build understanding, and develop strong tools for individuals to use moving forward to avoid or resolve future conflicts. Conflicts may arise from internal or external stressors and are further compounded within the healthcare sector by continually shifting priorities, differing perceptions and expectations, poor communication, and competition for resources.

Two techniques used to address conflict include conflict resolution and mediation. Both have goals of assisting the parties with finding common ground and formulating a plan to move forward in a manner that is professional and agreeable. Conflict resolution is achieved when the parties involved can communicate respectfully and compromise to seek a solution. Mediation may be used at any time in this process. This adds an additional party trained to facilitate conflict resolution. This individual does not have any stake in the conflict, provides guidance to allow for civil conversation, and provides a neutral perspective.

As a nurse, conflict is a common occurrence among staff, the multidisciplinary team, family, and even one's own internal morals or beliefs. The nurse may be involved in different roles during conflict, such as the mediator, participant, or observer. Facility policies will guide appropriate steps to follow when conflict has escalated, such as who to notify or include in escalating conflict. Examples include security,

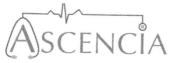

patient experience officers, or charge nurses. It is best to attempt to start with the lowest level of de-escalation techniques and safe practices and increase as the situation unfolds. As an example, a family member who is starting to become agitated may not need security involvement at the beginning. The nurse should be familiar with a variety of de-escalation techniques to employ to try to alleviate the situation prior to escalation.

Violence in healthcare settings has been steadily increasing over the past decade. De-escalation is a technique that all healthcare workers should have working knowledge of to prevent and reduce the frequency of violent behavior, avoid using restraints, increase patient satisfaction, and improve the safety of patients, the patient's family, and staff.

Many different types of assessments and tools can be applied to escalating behavior and situations including the Overt Aggression Scale; Broset Violence Checklist; and Assessment, Communication, and Tactics (ACT). There are some universal tenets in these tools that may be applied in most healthcare settings. These include creating a culture of safety with prominent displays that set expectations of a violence-free environment, providing mandatory de-escalation training for all staff, adopting a de-escalation model, and using debriefing techniques to improve future performance. Nurses may employ the use of early identification, creating a calm and noise-free environment, acknowledging tension and feelings, providing distractors or alternatives to current behavior, and supporting all parties.

Information Sharing

Situation, Background, Assessment, Recommendation (SBAR)

There will be many times that the nurse will need to update providers and other members of the healthcare team on the patient's condition. This information may be delivered in person, over the telephone, or by electronic messaging. It is important to ensure that the most important information is delivered clearly, effectively, and promptly and elicits the most beneficial response for the safety of the patient. The nurse will need to effectively report patient changes such as respiratory distress, hemodynamic instability, change in code status, reaction to a medication, unexpected response to treatment, or any other concern that the nurse needs the provider to address immediately or within a prompt timeframe.

To accomplish this, standardized tools have been developed to assist the nurse in ensuring that these goals are met. One such tool is called the SBAR (Situation-Background-Assessment-Recommendation). A standardized tool to enhance communication ensures that the most important information is shared between the sender and recipient, reducing the chances that pertinent information will be misunderstood or altogether missed in over-complication:

- *Situation* describes the exact nature of what is going on with the patient. Any non-essential information should be avoided and only the most important and pertinent details described. The nurse should clearly assign the severity of the situation to the audience during this introductory briefing.

- Next, the events leading up to the situation will be communicated. The *Background* will include the patient's diagnoses, reason for admission, medical history, and the unfolding patient picture that has led to this communication. In this section, abnormal vital signs and labs, current medications with last dosages, allergies, and any other clinically indicated information will be relayed.

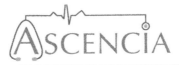

- During the *Assessment,* the nurse will relay the patient's current health status and nursing judgment of the reason the patient is experiencing the event. The nurse should provide the patient's current treatments, intravenous access sites, medication infusions, treatments provided (e.g., respiratory treatments), oxygenation supplementation required, input and output, and physical and mental observations.

- Finally, *Recommendations* are addressed. Experienced nurses may feel comfortable suggesting and requesting potential orders or treatment; however, the most important points to overtly communicate are what is required to improve the patient's condition, the urgency of the event, and what action must occur to address the patient's needs.

Prior to the nurse calling or approaching the provider, it is important to have information associated with the patient easily accessible. If possible, having the chart open to quickly refer to any information the provider may ask for is ideal; however, this may not always be accessible. At the minimum, the nurse should have on hand the following information: the patient's diagnosis, pertinent allergies, recent lab values, current and trends of vital signs, and any other clinical information related to the chief complaint. With any reporting tool, the nurse should first identify themselves, what unit or area the patient is in, and whether it is inpatient or outpatient. The name and date of birth of the patient should be stated upfront so that the provider may be provided with an early reference to identify and access the patient's chart.

Nursing Hand-Off Report

The nursing hand-off report is the opportunity for patient information to be communicated by the offgoing nurse to the oncoming nurse. This should occur at all instances of patient transfer of care, which may include acquiring a new caregiver due to a reassignment or shift change, changes in the level of care, or completing a facility-to-facility transfer. It is important to keep in mind that not all transfers denote an escalation of care. Patients being discharged from hospital care to long-term care still require a hand-off.

The hand-off should also include a verbal component. While electronic or paper hand-offs can help facilitate the hand-off process, the opportunity to discuss and clarify questions should be encouraged. The timing of the hand-off should coincide with the time that care will be transferred.

The minimal content that should be included in the patient hand-off are the critical components that are required to ensure care is safe and thorough. With facility transfers, the contact information of the sender should be given early on in case connection is lost. The current diagnosis (including severity) along with the current plan of care and treatment status must be understood by the receiver. A patient summary of the timeline of events, reason for clinical care, prior treatments, trends of assessments, timed vital signs and labs, allergy list, code status, and current medication list are the highest priority items to convey.

In an inpatient setting, the use of bedside reporting is recommended as best practice and has been adopted by facilities nationwide. This promotes patient-centered care as the patient is present for the report and updated to their plan of care and can contribute to the hand-off. The offgoing nurse can introduce the oncoming nurse directly to the patient. During this time, vital signs, labs, and IV infusions can be verified. Ideally, a computer workstation would be available at the patient's bedside. The focus is on communicating the information that is vital to ensuring that the patient may be safely cared for in a timely manner. When possible, it is best to include other members of the multidisciplinary team. Accomplishing this as a team provides time to consult, update, discuss, and ask and answer questions.

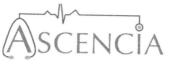

Barriers to an effective patient hand-off include incomplete or erroneous information, interruptions, incomplete documentation, poor communication, lack of standardization to reporting, limitations of time, insufficient staffing, disturbances of patient or family, and fear of not complying with HIPAA and divulging sensitive information.

These barriers may be overcome through a culture change that promotes and encourages a patient-centered, collaborative effort that involves management education and support. A standardized checklist has been found to improve compliance and consistency among nursing staff in adopting the bedside report practice.

Closed-Loop Communication

As a key component of thorough communication, the closed-loop communication model aims to ensure that both the sender and receiver are aligned in the message given and received. A method is utilized using callouts, check-backs, or read-backs to "close" the loop of communication.

The sender declares the message clearly and concisely. It is important that the message the sender is communicating is brief, focuses on one or two items, and is easily understood. The receiver accepts and processes the message, then confirms that the message was received with an affirmative statement, and the message is repeated back. This is the highly important check-back or read-back method. The sender then confirms that the information is accurate.

This is especially effective in ensuring that the correct message was conveyed and received when giving and receiving orders. This style of communication is highly relied upon in high-stress areas—emergency rooms, operating rooms, and critical care for code blue situations—but may be applied to any setting. It gives both parties the opportunity to verify and validate that the information is correct. Any questions or concerns may be addressed at that moment as well.

The applicability of closed-loop communication is highly reliable in cases where the message may be misheard or distorted. Verbal provider orders may be given in person but are more commonly received over the telephone. Many factors may prevent the receiver from understanding the message that the sender intended.

Verbal orders are particularly prone to misunderstandings and errors during the ordering process. Interruptions, background noise or static, enunciation, and complex or same-sounding drug names can cause interference in the message being received as intended. Using closed-loop communication for verbal orders allows the provider and the nurse a chance to verify that the order is correct.

Huddle

Frequently held at the start of a new shift or mid-shift, the huddle is used in healthcare as a brief meeting that communicates the plan for the day and creates situational awareness of unit assignments and the workflow of coworkers. Studies have shown that this improves teamwork and creates opportunities for improved relationships. Participants may include nurses, nursing assistants, charge nurses, and unit supervisors or managers as well as the interdisciplinary team including providers, therapists, clerks, and social workers.

The huddle should include important updates, staffing, patient census and acuity, care coordination, task delegation, and the discussion of any patient safety concerns. Patient concerns addressed may include changes in patient conditions, high-risk medications, fall alerts, disruptive behaviors, planning for anticipated admissions and discharges, and isolation precautions. This creates an opportunity to clarify any uncertainties and manage potential or anticipated crises prior to them occurring.

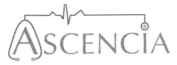

A tool that is growing in popularity is the use of a huddle board. This communication is usually placed in a prominent area where staff, patients, and visitors may see it. The purpose is to display a constantly evolving and perpetual update for the team. Included are staffing matrixes, patient census, assignments, daily and weekly updates, operational strategies, safety focuses, and unit and facility metrics.

Interdisciplinary Communication

Interdisciplinary healthcare teams communicate over a variety of mediums for different purposes. This communication may be informal, such as face-to-face casual talk, impromptu conversations in hallways, notes left on charts or with the personal belongings of the receiver, and even within computerized messaging systems. Informal conversations can cover a broad number of topics from reminders to provide family with updates, calling another healthcare team member, discussion of topics of common interest, sharing patient or organizational information, and concerns or questions that may have healthcare relevance but are not directly tied to a certain patient or situation. While informal interdisciplinary communication is a common practice, the nurse must also ensure compliance with HIPAA regulations.

Formal communication tends to be scheduled and focused on a topic or patient care function. This may be informational or educational. The goal is to create a cohesive team that is informed and able to synergistically work together as a unit to accomplish a goal.

During educational meetings, subject matter experts are often utilized to present content. These may be members of the interdisciplinary team or outside sources, such as medical equipment or pharmaceutical representatives. This form of communication is also used to deliver information, such as administrative announcements, to an individual or a wide audience. These may be delivered orally in person, via pre-recorded video, or by written letter.

Communication Barriers

Language Barriers

When a patient is not fluent in the language primarily used within a facility, patient care can suffer. In the United States, this is usually the limited ability to speak, write, or understand the English language. To achieve patient-centered care, the nurse must ensure that the patient can freely communicate, actively participate in conversation, and have a mutual understanding of their care plan. All patients with limited English proficiency who are receiving federal assistance (with the exception of Medicare Part B) that have patient care services provided at healthcare clinics or facilities must be offered the opportunity to participate in a translating service. This rule is in accordance with Title VI of the Civil Rights Act. This is best practice to extend to all patients who are not fluent in the English language.

Translating services include trained bilingual caregivers, licensed in-person translators, and telephone and video conference services. These translating services are often contracted by the organization and may require advance notice to accommodate. Facility policy should dictate the translation services available, how to schedule the service, and pertinent contact information. Some healthcare providers may also be specially trained to provide interpretation services.

If an interpreter is not available, the family may be used to translate; however, certain guidelines should be adhered to. The family member must be fluent in English and the native language of the patient and be over eighteen years of age. Most importantly, the patient must have agreed to this arrangement. In cases of emergency, following these guidelines may not be possible, and critical thinking should evaluate risk versus benefits.

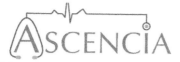

Hearing Impairments

When a patient has a hearing impairment, augmentative and alternative communication devices are available to enhance communication. These include picture boards or electronic touch screens displaying commonly used shapes or words to illustrate meaning. Devices used should be based on the level of the patient's education, dexterity, and familiarity of use.

When communication or education is delivered via video, the nurse should assess the patient's access to resources that can improve delivery tailored to the patient's needs. The level of hearing impairment may need a different approach. There are assistive devices, such as amplifiers, that improve sound quality and reduce background noises. Many types are available, including frequency-modulator systems, infrared systems, and hearing loop systems. Additional equipment may be required with some of these devices. Another available tool is closed captioning. This service is readily available on most electronic devices and turns spoken words into text that scrolls across the screen.

As with all education delivered to the patient, the nurse must follow up to ensure understanding. When a patient has any sensory deficit or impairment, this is especially challenging. It is best practice to be at the patient's bedside when providers are updating or teaching patients so that it is known what has been communicated and to facilitate communication. If the nurse did not have the opportunity to be present, the provider should be contacted to verify the education provided. The nurse should then allow the patient to teach back what their understanding was. Assistive devices and communication tools should be encouraged to promote understanding. Family or friends, with the patient's permission, can help by reiterating the education provided and also providing a secondary source for reminders.

Visual Impairments

Visual impairment may range from blurred vision to color blindness to full blindness. It can also be a result of multiple conditions. Some patients may require minimal aid while others rely fully upon assistive technology. There is a wide variety of assistive hardware and software available that can give broader access to communication and interaction with technology. One of the most prevalent software types available is text-to-speech software. This technology enables blind or visually impaired individuals to utilize computers as well as to turn scanned printed material into an audio format. Screen readers are available that produce a readable braille output. Braille is a form of language that is made up of a series of dots that can be translated via touch. There are also refreshable braille screens that use software and hardware to display braille pins that electronically raise and lower.

Cognitive Impairments

Cognition is the mental capacity to acquire knowledge and develop thoughts through the processing of high-level intellectual functions including, but not limited to, decision-making, planning, judgment, language, memory, and attention. There is a broad range of cognitive impairments that may be acute or chronic. Each requires a distinct and specific style of communication tactics to ensure the best possible communication with the individual. The nature of each type of cognitive disorder and how it affects each facet of cognitive performance must be considered to deliver communication that facilitates the patient functioning at their highest level.

Cognitive disorders are marked by the inability to function in society without treatment. Alzheimer's disease is the disorder most associated with cognitive impairment. However, there are an array of disorders and conditions, such as hypoglycemia, autism, malnutrition, heavy metal disease, delirium,

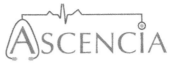

dementia, depression, substance abuse, schizophrenic disorders, and prion disease, that contribute to early and late cognitive deficits.

Each of these requires a tailored approach based on both the specific patient and disease process. Disorders such as Alzheimer's require patience and time to process thoughts as individuals are often withdrawn. These individuals may have difficulties with speech and forming logical or linear thoughts, and they may rely upon gestures to try to connect. In these cases, it is better to use questions that are direct and only require a yes or no answer. In contrast, disorders that cause impulsivity issues, outbursts, and difficulty concentrating, such as ADHD in children, may require interaction that is very concise, uses gestures, and enunciates clearly. Having the child restate what was communicated once their full attention is gained can improve understanding and interactivity.

Critical Thinking

Time Management and Prioritization of Care

Time management is a critical part of providing competent and safe patient care. The nurse will have to deal with multiple priorities and challenges at different times of the day and must formulate a plan to deal with both higher acuity concerns as well as ensure that the standard of care is met for patients who do not require urgent care. Specific time management habits will increase the probability of success. These include planning and goal setting, prioritizing care, and seeking out ways that will decrease the amount of time spent on individual tasks.

At the start of the shift, a strategy may be to first identify the most important tasks that are the nurse's responsibility to complete, with a triage of top priorities that must be completed throughout the day. A hierarchy of care should be established based on patient acuity, any scheduled procedures, timeliness to complete tasks, and potential for harm. Priorities of care are determined by assessments focused respectively on airway, breathing, and circulation.

Next, any duties that may be delegated should be planned with the individual who will carry out the actions. Delegation is integral to the workflow of the nursing unit and should be used to the utmost advantage. The decision to delegate should be based on a set of standards, including the patient's acuity level, the availability of the staff being delegated to, and the level and complexity of supervision required. Nurses must be cognizant of who they are delegating to, ensure that the right person is assigned to the right task, and oversee results. It is the responsibility of the nurse to assess that the person being assigned a task is competent and has experience with the task or assignment being delegated.

Clustering care is a major move to decrease inefficiencies in patient care. Some prior planning is required to make this work both effectively and efficiently. Essentially, it is doing as much care for the patient at one time as possible. When giving medications, the patient may need toileting or a wound dressing change. These are all done at the same time rather than spreading them throughout the day. It is important to always check whether the patient requires anything else prior to leaving the room to avoid being called back in a few minutes.

Establishing routines is another strategy that can set the precedence for how each day is managed. By creating a process that establishes a set of habits, the nurse can diminish the loss of time by eliminating the planning factor.

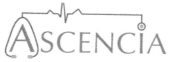

Many organizations are moving towards implementing strategies that reduce the number of interruptions to nurses. Interruptions are a significant time waster and increase the risk of patient harm. Creating "quiet zones" or "no interruption zones," especially surrounding medication administration tasks, is a way to allow nurses to focus on the task, improve safety, and reduce interruptions that lead to delays in patient care. These may be marked via red tape or a vest that the nurse wears while occupied by the task. This visual reminder gives a cautionary warning for others not to impede the safety of the nurse or the patients.

Teamwork is essential to ensure safe patient care is provided regardless of the healthcare environment. Organizations must foster trust, reliance, professional development, and a culture of safety. With the increasing complexity of patient care, communication, camaraderie, and acting as a collective unit are essential in fully embracing patient-centered care. When each team member knows their role and contributes to the multidisciplinary healthcare team, the interdependent knowledge and skills provide a patient with a well-rounded, coordinated care experience.

Crisis Management and Resources

Nurses must care for patients in all stages of illness and health. At times, without warning, a patient's health status can quickly decline. When this occurs, backup healthcare assistance is a way to support the nurse assigned to the patient and provide expert guidance. A decline in patient status may be marked by changes in airway, breathing, or circulation. Audible gasping, vital signs that are outside of normal measures, syncopal episodes, and dysrhythmias are all common signs of clinical deterioration.

Organizations may create a team that is trained to respond to such circumstances. This is often referred to as a "rapid response team." This interdisciplinary team varies depending on the size of the organization and acuity of the patient population and may have different models based on the type of clinical emergency. A simple rapid-response team is typically composed of a charge nurse or critical care nurse, a respiratory therapist, and a physician (hospitalist or specialist). Another form of the rapid response team is a critical outreach team. This is meant to provide guidance to manage a situation prior to severe patient deterioration and may be a physician and critical care nurse. Finally, a medical emergency team is formed to immediately respond to active emergencies such as a code blue (respiratory or cardiac arrest).

These teams may serve in different capacities, but their duties are similar. Responding and providing advanced care to patient emergencies is the priority. These teams may also provide guidance for critical care patients transitioning to step-down care. This type of guidance includes proactive evaluation and assessment of patients identified to have a high risk for certain conditions and educating unit staff on the best practices to manage such patients. These teams may also act in a consultative manner with patients who require a higher level of care due to a condition or diagnosis but who are not in crisis.

A patient's condition may rapidly decline, but often there are subtle signs leading up to the clinical crisis. Being aware of the patient's history, the pathophysiology of diagnosis, the expected response from current treatment, and being in tune with the nuances that may suggest that the patient's progress is not as expected can all provide warning signs for the nurse to be attuned to. When vital signs and assessments start to show changes that are not physiologic, the nurse should focus on employing interventions to support the patient's functional status. The nurse should be aware of ordered medications to be administered based on parameters, standing orders, or facility protocol to manage potential health emergencies such as hypoglycemia, bradycardia, hypo- or hypertension, or allergic reactions. Immediately upon concern of a patient declining, the nurse should request assistance from colleagues. This may be another nurse or a charge nurse. The nurse caring for the patient should not

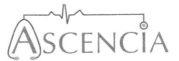

leave the bedside unless it is unavoidable. Guidance may be gained from other perspectives. If the nurse is unsure whether the patient is having a crisis but there is a concern, requesting the opinion from another unit that manages that type of condition is helpful. Always notify the healthcare provider immediately when there are significant changes in the patient's condition. The rapid response team is not only there to respond to active crises but also for additional support. With any indecisiveness regarding the patient's condition or a different level of acuity from what the med-surg nurse is competent in, the rapid response team may be consulted.

Critical Thinking

Personal bias can be a barrier to fair and equitable patient care when it allows personal opinions, thoughts, and beliefs to influence judgment and actions. This results in an environment that does not support the needs of a patient, group, or community. Bias may be directed towards any aspect of an individual or group. These aspects include race, age, sex, sexual orientation, culture, religion, drug dependency, weight, or affluence.

Explicit bias is overt and known. These are thoughts and actions directed purposefully towards a group due to upbringing, norms, policies, or accepted practices. These attitudes, beliefs, and tendencies can easily be self-identified and are commonly endorsed, communicated, and consistent throughout an individual's reflection of self. Racist comments are a common form of explicit bias. Other types of explicit biases include sexual harassment, unfair pay based on sex or race, and promotions or work assignments based on favoritism.

Implicit bias is an unconscious, unrealized stereotype or belief that shapes opinions, decisions, actions, and understanding of the community. The individual who is exhibiting these biases is unaware of their projection or the damage it may cause. Unlike stereotyping—which makes broad, negative assumptions or views about a group, culture, or category of individuals—implicit bias can be both favorable or unfavorable and guide the decision-making process.

Through the use of critical thinking skills, nurses must be aware of both explicit and implicit biases and confront the potential harm they may cause with patient care. A self-assessment is an excellent method of identifying bias that may be overt or underlying. Over the last several years, organizations have been actively tackling bias via education, policy, and cultural change. Some states have enforced the requirement of continued education in implicit bias and inclusivity for healthcare providers. Utilizing these resources will allow the nurse to understand the harm that bias does to patient care, identify the different types of bias that are prevalent within the healthcare system and community, and describe best practices to advocate for patient care that promotes equitable healthcare.

Clinical decisions are best supported by critical thinking. Nurses are trained to follow a systematic and methodical process: ADPIE (Assess-Diagnose-Plan-Intervene-Evaluate). This paradigm provides a method to analytically evaluate clinical signs and patient presentation that leads to evidence-based judgments. Initially, an analysis of the patient is provided through a thorough assessment and consideration of the patient's history and current care plan. This observed data can be interpreted via the working knowledge gained through education, experience, and deference to expert advice and opinion. Inferences are made and guided by weighing data against logic and reasoning. Critical thinking is built over time and experience; however, following the nursing model will help build the ability to effectively problem solve and begin to recognize the standards and characteristics that lead to appropriate conclusions.

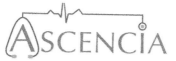

The nurse will use this map to guide decision-making throughout each patient encounter. It may be applied to high acuity, critical situations as well as standard processes.

The critical thinking process is applied to the following case study:

0700 - A nurse is caring for a patient with a history of syncopal episodes. The patient is currently on telemetry, and the screen alarms that the patient is bradycardic. The nurse evaluates the monitor and checks on the patient. The patient is sitting up in bed, alert and oriented, and states comfort. A palpable pulse confirms that the pulse is 35 beats per minute. The nurse reviews the MAR for 0700 medications and notes that metoprolol tartrate 25 mg is due. How can the nurse apply critical thinking to this situation?

Based on the mechanism of action of metoprolol tartrate as a beta blocker, this medication lowers heart rate. The nurse recognizes that this is a probable cause of the bradycardia and that administering at this time may decrease the heart rate even lower. Inferred judgment via critical thinking leads the nurse to hold the medication until consulting with the physician regarding a lower dose or a different medication.

Healthy Practice Environment

Workplace Safety

Physical and Environmental Workplace Safety

Physical and environmental workplace safety is of paramount importance in the healthcare industry, particularly in nursing practice. It encompasses various aspects, such as ensuring safe equipment, proper disposal of sharps and biohazardous materials, and maintaining adequate lighting. Additionally, having sufficient physical resources, including functional equipment and appropriate staffing levels, is crucial for providing high-quality patient care.

Safe equipment is essential for preventing accidents and injuries among both healthcare providers and patients. Regular maintenance and inspections help ensure that medical devices and tools are in proper working condition. Adequate lighting is necessary for accurate assessment, medication administration, and surgical procedures, as poor lighting can lead to errors and compromised patient safety.

Proper disposal of sharps and biohazardous materials is vital in preventing the spread of infections and protecting the environment. Healthcare facilities must adhere to strict guidelines for the safe disposal of such materials to minimize the risk of contamination.

Furthermore, having the right physical resources, including safe equipment and adequate staffing, plays a critical role in maintaining patient safety and delivering effective care. Safe and functional equipment helps healthcare providers perform their tasks efficiently, and adequate staffing and nurse-to-patient ratios ensure that patients receive the attention and care they need without compromising quality or safety.

In summary, physical and environmental workplace safety in nursing practice involves ensuring safe equipment, proper disposal of hazardous materials, and adequate resources. These measures are essential for safeguarding the well-being of both healthcare providers and patients.

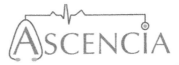

Emotional Workplace Safety

Emotional workplace safety is a critical aspect of nursing practice that goes beyond physical well-being, encompassing the psychological and emotional well-being of healthcare professionals. It is characterized by a workplace culture where staff members feel comfortable asking questions, requesting changes, and expressing their opinions without fear of reprisal or judgment.

Nurse resiliency is a central component of emotional workplace safety. It refers to a nurse's ability to adapt and bounce back from various challenges encountered in the healthcare setting. This includes the capacity to cope with a stressful shift, navigate conflicts with colleagues or patients, and embrace change, such as floating to a different unit when necessary. Resilient nurses can maintain their composure, continue providing high-quality care, and support their peers during challenging times.

Adaptability in the workplace is crucial for responding to the dynamic nature of healthcare. Nurses often face situations where they must step out of their comfort zones, such as working in unfamiliar units. Adaptability ensures that nurses can provide effective care, regardless of the circumstances.

Furthermore, peer accountability plays a pivotal role in improving the emotional workplace environment. This concept encourages nurses to hold themselves and their colleagues accountable for personal growth and team development. It fosters a collaborative atmosphere where constructive feedback is valued, ultimately enhancing emotional workplace safety by promoting open communication and mutual support among healthcare professionals.

Unintended Consequences

An unhealthy workplace environment in healthcare can result in significant consequences for professionals. Moral distress and moral injuries occur when healthcare providers perceive a conflict between their ethical values and workplace demands, leading to emotional anguish and potential trauma. Burnout is characterized by emotional exhaustion, depersonalization, and reduced personal accomplishment, primarily due to chronic workplace stress. Compassion fatigue arises when caregivers become emotionally drained from consistently providing empathy and support, potentially leading to reduced compassion and increased rates of errors in patient care. These consequences underscore the importance of addressing workplace issues, promoting staff well-being, and providing support to healthcare professionals to ensure not only their own mental and emotional health but also the quality of care they deliver to patients.

Scope of Practice and Ethics

Nursing Scope and Standards of Practice

The Academy of Medical-Surgical Nurses (AMSN) Scope and Standards of Practice provides a vital framework that outlines the nursing role in delivering patient-centered interventions, taking into consideration the patient's preferences and choices as a priority. Nurses play a crucial role in ensuring that interventions are not only evidence-based but also aligned with the patient's goals and values. This involves respecting the patient's autonomy, preferences, and informed choices, even when those choices might differ from the nurse's recommendations.

The AMSN Scope and Standards of Practice underscores the nurse's responsibility to advocate for the patient's well-being, ensuring that interventions are not imposed but rather collaboratively decided

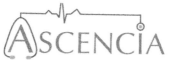

upon with the patient. Nurses are encouraged to engage in effective communication and shared decision-making, fostering a partnership with the patient in their care journey.

Moreover, these standards highlight the necessity of providing culturally competent and ethical care. Nurses should consider the patient's cultural background and values when planning and delivering interventions, further respecting the patient's unique perspective and preferences.

In essence, the AMSN Scope and Standards of Practice reinforces the pivotal role of medical-surgical nurses in advocating for patient well-being by providing interventions that align with the patient's wishes, values, and goals, ultimately ensuring patient-centered care and the highest standards of practice.

Nursing Code of Ethics

The Nursing Code of Ethics serves as a foundational framework that guides the ethical behavior and professional conduct of nurses. At its core, it underscores the nursing role as a patient advocate, with the primary goal of providing high-quality patient care while upholding the principles of dignified and respectful patient care.

Patient advocacy is a central tenet of nursing ethics. Nurses are entrusted with the responsibility of ensuring that the patients' best interests are paramount in all healthcare decisions and actions. This advocacy includes safeguarding patient autonomy, promoting informed consent, and facilitating open and honest communication between patients and healthcare teams. Nurses are not only caregivers but also educators and supporters, empowering patients to make informed choices about their healthcare.

The Nursing Code of Ethics provides nurses with a set of guiding principles, often organized into a framework with interpretive standards. These standards outline the ethical obligations and responsibilities that nurses must uphold in their practice. They cover areas such as respect for human dignity, patient confidentiality, professional boundaries, and the duty to provide competent and safe care.

One notable example of a nursing code of ethics is the American Nurses Association (ANA) Code of Ethics for Nurses with Interpretive Statements. This code comprises nine provisions that offer ethical guidance and set expectations for nurses. Interpretive statements further clarify each provision, providing practical examples and considerations for nurses in various practice settings.

In summary, the Nursing Code of Ethics highlights the crucial role of nurses as patient advocates, emphasizing the provision of quality care while preserving the dignity and rights of patients. It offers a comprehensive framework, such as the Code of Ethics for Nurses with Interpretive Statements, to guide nurses in making ethically sound decisions and maintaining the highest standards of professional conduct in their daily practice.

Patients' Rights and Responsibilities

Patients' rights and responsibilities are foundational principles in healthcare that promote mutual respect, ethical treatment, and effective communication between patients and healthcare providers. Patients have the right to receive high-quality care that respects their dignity and autonomy. This includes the right to informed consent, privacy, confidentiality, and access to their medical records. Patients also have the right to voice grievances and participate in decisions about their care.

In tandem with these rights, patients also bear responsibilities, such as providing accurate medical information, following recommended treatment plans, and treating healthcare providers and staff with

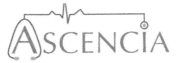

respect and courtesy. Patients should also be actively engaged in their healthcare, ask questions, and seek clarifications when needed. By upholding these rights and responsibilities, a collaborative and patient-centered approach to healthcare can be achieved, ultimately promoting the well-being and satisfaction of patients and improving the quality of care they receive.

Recognizing and Reporting Unethical Practice

In healthcare, recognizing and reporting unethical practices is vital in ensuring patient safety, maintaining professional integrity, and upholding the highest standards of care. Self-regulation practices play a crucial role in identifying and addressing unethical behaviors and situations within the healthcare environment.

One common area of concern is unsafe staffing levels, which can compromise patient care quality and safety. Healthcare professionals have a responsibility to recognize when staffing levels are inadequate to provide safe care and to report these concerns to appropriate authorities or supervisors.

Practicing outside the scope of practice is another unethical behavior that healthcare professionals must vigilantly monitor. Each healthcare discipline has a defined scope of practice, and each discipline should not perform tasks or procedures beyond their authorized role. Recognizing and reporting instances where individuals are exceeding their scope helps protect patient safety and maintain professional boundaries.

Furthermore, healthcare professionals must be vigilant about unsafe practice facilities, such as environments with inadequate infection control measures or safety protocols. Identifying and reporting these issues is essential for preventing harm to both patients and healthcare workers.

In summary, self-regulation practices in healthcare encompass identifying concerns related to unsafe staffing, healthcare professionals operating outside their scope of practice, and unsafe practice facilities. By actively recognizing and reporting these ethical breaches, healthcare professionals uphold their duty to provide high-quality, safe care and contribute to a culture of accountability and ethical conduct in healthcare settings.

Policies, Procedures, and Regulatory Requirements

Policies, procedures, and regulatory requirements serve as fundamental guidelines that ensure the provision of safe, effective, and ethical healthcare. Various entities, including professional organizations, federal agencies, state bodies, and individual healthcare facilities, play pivotal roles in establishing and enforcing these regulations and standards.

Professional organizations, such as the ANA, are influential in shaping the standards of practice and ethical guidelines for healthcare professionals. The ANA develops the Nursing Code of Ethics, a foundational document that guides nurses in their moral and professional obligations, emphasizing patient-centered care and ethical conduct. These standards help maintain the integrity and quality of nursing practice.

Federal regulations are a cornerstone of healthcare governance in the United States. Bodies like the Joint Commission and Centers for Medicare & Medicaid Services (CMS) are responsible for establishing and overseeing healthcare standards. The Joint Commission accredits healthcare organizations, ensuring that they adhere to rigorous safety and quality standards. CMS, on the other hand, administers critical federal healthcare programs, setting regulations that impact reimbursement, quality measurement, and patient safety in facilities that accept Medicare and Medicaid funding.

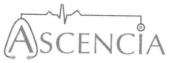

State regulations are another crucial layer of healthcare governance. Each state has a Board of Nursing that enforces the Nurse Practice Act. This Act defines the scope of nursing practice, licensure requirements, and standards of care. State nursing boards grant and regulate nursing licenses, ensuring that nurses practice within their state's legal and ethical boundaries.

Within healthcare facilities and agencies, specific policies, procedures, and protocols further shape clinical practice. These documents provide detailed instructions for various aspects of care, from infection control measures to medication administration protocols. Adherence to facility-specific policies and procedures is essential for maintaining consistency, safety, and quality of care within the organization.

In conclusion, policies, procedures, and regulatory requirements are essential components of the healthcare landscape. They are established and upheld by various entities, including professional organizations, federal agencies, state nursing boards, and individual healthcare facilities. These regulations and standards are designed to safeguard patient well-being, maintain the integrity of the nursing profession, and ensure that healthcare services are provided with the utmost quality, ethics, and safety. Nurses play a vital role in understanding and adhering to these guidelines in order to provide optimal care and maintain compliance with the ever-evolving landscape of healthcare regulations.

Quality Management

Nursing Sensitive Indicators

Nursing-Sensitive Indicators (NSIs) play a pivotal role in measuring the quality of nursing care and its impact on patient outcomes. The National Database of Nursing Quality Indicators (NDNQI), formulated by the American Nurses Association (ANA), stands as an up-to-date and comprehensive resource for tracking and analyzing these indicators, providing valuable insights into the effectiveness of nursing practice.

Adverse events, such as falls and nosocomial infections, are key NSIs that directly reflect the quality of nursing care. Falls can result in injuries and complications, and nosocomial infections, which are acquired in healthcare settings, can lead to prolonged hospital stays and increased healthcare costs. By monitoring these indicators, healthcare institutions can identify areas of vulnerability and implement preventive measures, ultimately enhancing patient safety.

Nursing satisfaction records are equally significant NSIs, as they provide insights into nurses' job satisfaction and engagement. High nurse satisfaction is often associated with better patient care outcomes, lower turnover rates, and improved patient experiences. In evolving nursing practice models, ensuring nursing satisfaction is essential for retaining skilled professionals and maintaining the continuity of care.

Staffing models, including nurse-to-patient ratios, are critical NSIs that significantly impact patient care. Appropriate staffing levels are essential for providing safe and effective care. Inadequate staffing can lead to burnout, increased stress, and decreased job satisfaction among nurses, which can negatively affect patient care quality. Monitoring staffing models through NSIs ensures that these models are optimized to provide the best possible patient care.

These quality indicators are crucial for evolving nursing practice models for several reasons. Firstly, they enable healthcare organizations to make data-driven decisions, leading to improved patient outcomes

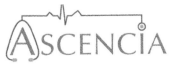

and enhanced nursing practice. Secondly, they help identify areas of improvement, allowing nurses and healthcare institutions to focus on evidence-based interventions to enhance care quality. Thirdly, NSIs support the evaluation of the impact of evolving practice models, ensuring that changes lead to positive outcomes for both patients and nurses.

In summary, NSIs are vital components of modern healthcare quality measurement. The NDNQI, formulated by the ANA, serves as a valuable resource for tracking and analyzing these indicators, providing insights into nursing care quality. As nursing practice models continue to evolve, NSIs will remain essential tools for optimizing patient care, enhancing nursing satisfaction, and achieving positive patient outcomes.

Quality Assurance and Performance Improvement

Quality Assurance (QA) and Performance Improvement (PI) are integral components of healthcare delivery, extending across both inpatient and outpatient settings. These dynamic processes are continuous in nature, reflecting the commitment to maintaining and enhancing healthcare quality.

QA programs serve as structured mechanisms for monitoring and assessing care quality, embracing a proactive approach to identifying areas of concern, and mitigating deviations from established standards. Whether in inpatient or outpatient settings, QA teams play a pivotal role in recognizing patterns, preventing recurring issues, and ensuring patient safety while upholding clinical excellence.

One of the outcomes of an active QA program is the initiation of PI projects. These projects emerge from the thorough analysis of QA findings, pinpointing specific areas that require enhancement. Stakeholders from various disciplines collaborate in PI projects to implement evidence-based interventions, with the overarching goal of elevating patient and clinical satisfaction. These initiatives extend beyond addressing patient outcomes and workflow efficiency; they encompass an array of factors that contribute to a positive healthcare experience.

The roles of QA/PI teams are multifaceted, encompassing responsibilities such as investigating occurrences, conducting root cause analyses, identifying areas for improvement, and collaborating with multidisciplinary teams. Their efforts foster a culture of continuous improvement, ensuring that healthcare practices evolve in response to shifting patient needs and are aligned with the latest clinical evidence. As healthcare continually advances, the dedication to QA and PI remains a cornerstone of providing high-quality, patient-centered care.

Nursing Professional Practice Model

A Nursing Professional Practice Model serves as a foundational framework that guides nursing practice within healthcare facilities. This comprehensive model encompasses several critical subtopics, including core professional values, professional relationships, recognition and compensation, care delivery systems, and management/administration principles. Together, these elements shape the philosophy and approach to nursing care:

- Core Professional Values: At the core of the Nursing Professional Practice Model are essential values such as compassion, integrity, respect, and advocacy. These values serve as the ethical foundation for nursing practice, guiding nurses in their interactions with patients, families, and colleagues.

- Professional Relationships: Effective communication and collaboration are vital for healthcare teams. Building strong professional relationships within nursing teams,

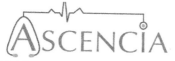

across interdisciplinary groups, and with patients and families fosters a positive work environment and enhances the quality of patient care.

- Recognition and Compensation: Recognizing nurses for their valuable contributions and ensuring fair compensation are crucial components of the model. Acknowledging nurses' dedication, expertise, and hard work not only motivates and retains high-quality nursing staff but also recognizes their pivotal role in patient care.

- Care Delivery Systems: This subtopic addresses how patient care is organized and delivered within the facility. It emphasizes the importance of efficient and patient-centered care delivery models, ensuring that care remains consistent, aligned with best practices, and focused on the patient's well-being.

- Management and Administration: Effective leadership and management principles provide the necessary support, guidance, and resources for frontline nurses. This subtopic outlines the roles and responsibilities of nursing leaders and administrators in creating a supportive work environment conducive to professional growth.

The Nursing Professional Practice Model is essential for the following reasons:

- Quality and Consistency: It sets clear standards for nursing practice, ensuring a consistent approach to care delivery, enhancing patient safety, and quality.

- Alignment With Goals: It aligns nursing practice with the facility's mission, ensuring that care reflects organizational objectives.

- Job Satisfaction: Nurses within this model often experience higher job satisfaction due to role clarity and support.

- Patient Experience: Patients benefit from care that emphasizes values, relationships, and efficiency, resulting in a positive experience.

- Professional Growth: The model supports nurses' development, recognition, and advancement, fostering a skilled and engaged workforce.

A Nursing Professional Practice Model is fundamental, promoting ethical values, collaboration, recognition, efficient care, and management support. This framework ensures high-quality care, job satisfaction, positive patient experiences, and professional growth for nurses within healthcare facilities.

Adverse Event Reporting

Adverse event reporting is essential in healthcare to ensure patient safety and improve overall care quality. It involves defining adverse events, recognizing common types, and understanding the role of reporting in ensuring proper follow-up and driving quality QA and PI efforts.

Adverse events encompass unintended and harmful incidents occurring during medical care. These events range from medication errors to patient falls, equipment malfunctions, and nosocomial infections. They can result in patient harm, prolonged hospital stays, and increased healthcare costs.

Several prevalent types of adverse events pose significant risks to patient safety:

- Medication errors: These occur during prescribing, dispensing, administering, or monitoring medications, potentially leading to adverse drug reactions or inadequate treatment.

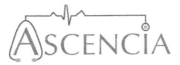

- Patient falls: Falls within healthcare settings can cause injuries, fractures, or complications, particularly among elderly or vulnerable patients.

- Equipment errors: Malfunctioning or improperly used medical equipment can compromise patient safety, delay treatment, or cause harm.

- Nosocomial infections: These infections develop during a patient's hospital stay and can result from various factors, including inadequate hand hygiene or insufficient infection control practices.

Reporting adverse events is crucial for several reasons:

- Prompt follow-up: Reporting facilitates immediate actions to address incidents, provide necessary care, and prevent further harm or complications.

- Quality assurance/performance improvement: It is integral to healthcare QA and PI initiatives. It helps identify areas needing improvement, implement preventive measures, and enhance patient safety.

- Legal and ethical obligations: Healthcare providers have legal and ethical responsibilities to report adverse events, upholding professional standards and ensuring patients' rights to proper care and compensation when necessary.

Patient/Customer Experience Based on Data Results

The patient/customer experience is a pivotal aspect of healthcare, emphasizing patient-centered care and continuous improvement. Healthcare facilities employ various methods to gauge and enhance this experience, such as surveys like the Hospital Consumer Assessment of Healthcare Providers and Systems (HCAHPS) and participation in value-based purchasing programs. These mechanisms allow facilities to gather valuable feedback and make data-driven improvements.

The "5 C's" framework is a guiding principle for delivering an exceptional patient/customer experience:

- Consistency: Patients value reliable care and communication. Ensuring consistency in treatment, information sharing, and service delivery instills a sense of trust and reliability in the healthcare system.

- Coordination: Effective coordination among different healthcare providers and departments is paramount. When patients perceive seamless transitions and collaborative efforts among their care team, it not only enhances their overall experience but also reduces confusion and frustration.

- Continuity: Maintaining ongoing, consistent relationships between patients and their healthcare providers fosters a better understanding of medical history, preferences, and unique needs, contributing to a positive and personalized experience.

- Caring: Empathy and compassion play a pivotal role in patient-centered care. Patients want to feel cared for as individuals, not merely as medical cases. Healthcare providers who demonstrate genuine concern for their patients' well-being have a profound impact on the overall experience.

- Correction: Acknowledging and rectifying errors or issues that arise in healthcare is essential. Swift and transparent correction of problems can salvage the patient experience, rebuild trust, and demonstrate the facility's commitment to improvement.

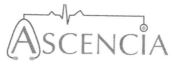

Elevating the patient/customer experience goes beyond ensuring patient satisfaction. It positively influences clinical outcomes. Satisfied patients are more likely to adhere to treatment plans, actively engage in their care, and maintain ongoing relationships with healthcare providers. Additionally, a positive patient experience contributes to better patient retention and can result in favorable word-of-mouth recommendations, ultimately benefiting the facility's reputation and community standing.

Service Recovery

Service recovery is a fundamental aspect of healthcare delivery aimed at restoring trust and confidence between patients and the healthcare team. It encompasses a strategic approach to addressing and resolving issues that may arise during the course of patient care. The overarching goal of service recovery is to acknowledge and rectify these issues promptly, ensuring that patients feel valued, heard, and cared for throughout their healthcare journey.

The process of service recovery typically involves several key steps:

- Recognition of the issue: Healthcare providers must be vigilant in recognizing when issues or concerns emerge. Whether it's a breakdown in communication, an unexpected outcome, or a delay in care, identifying the problem is the initial step.

- Issue resolution: Once identified, healthcare teams work collaboratively to address and resolve the issue. This may involve immediate corrective actions, changes in care plans, or additional support to meet the patient's needs.

- Follow-up: After the issue has been addressed, it's essential to follow up with the patient to ensure that their concerns have been adequately addressed and that they are satisfied with the actions taken. This step reinforces the commitment to patient-centered care.

- Follow-through: Service recovery extends beyond the immediate resolution of the issue. Healthcare providers should continuously monitor the situation, implement preventive measures, and make necessary improvements to prevent similar issues in the future.

Service recovery is not only about resolving problems but also about rebuilding trust and confidence in healthcare teams. When handled effectively, it can lead to stronger patient-provider relationships, improved patient satisfaction, and enhanced overall healthcare quality. By recognizing issues, taking swift action, following up with patients, and consistently following through on improvements, healthcare organizations can uphold their commitment to patient-centered care and ensure a positive patient experience.

Project Development

Project development follows a structured model comprising five phases—initiation, planning, execution, monitoring/controlling, and closing—that provide a road map for effective project management in various domains, including healthcare:

- Initiation: The project begins with initiation, where stakeholders identify its purpose, scope, objectives, and initial constraints. In healthcare, this may involve recognizing opportunities for improving patient care processes or implementing new technologies.

- Planning: In the planning phase, project managers (with input from the team and stakeholders) detail project objectives, scope, schedule, budget, and required

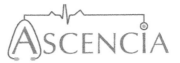

resources. Healthcare projects must align with quality and regulatory standards and ensure uninterrupted patient care.

- Execution: Execution translates the project plan into action. In healthcare, this could entail implementing new clinical protocols, adopting electronic health record systems, or facility renovations. Effective communication, resource allocation, and teamwork are essential to ensure smooth execution.

- Monitoring/Controlling: This phase runs alongside execution, involving continuous oversight and control of project activities. In healthcare, it includes tracking patient outcomes, resource use, and adherence to timelines. It enables early issue identification and corrective actions to maintain project alignment.

- Closing: Closing formalizes the project's conclusion. In healthcare, it encompasses finalizing patient care processes, assessing the project's impact, and ensuring a seamless transition to new systems. Lessons learned are documented, and successes are celebrated.

Evidence-Based Practice and Research

Legislative and licensure requirements play a pivotal role in governing evidence-based practice (EBP) and clinical research within the healthcare field. Understanding the distinctions between EBP and clinical research is fundamental, and healthcare professionals must be diligent in referring to their state board of nursing for specific legislative and licensure requirements.

EBP involves the integration of clinical expertise, patient values and preferences, and the best available evidence in healthcare decision-making. It aims to provide the most effective and safe care to patients, with the foundation of practice resting on current research and clinical guidelines.

Clinical research, on the other hand, focuses on the systematic investigation of healthcare interventions, treatments, or practices to generate new knowledge, validate existing evidence, or explore novel therapies. It often involves conducting experiments, clinical trials, and studies to gather data and draw conclusions that can inform medical practice.

Referring to the state board of nursing is crucial due to the variations in legislative and licensure requirements across different states. These boards establish and enforce the rules and regulations that govern the practice of nursing within their jurisdiction. This includes setting standards for EBP, clinical research, and other aspects of nursing practice.

The importance of consulting the state board of nursing lies in ensuring compliance with legal and professional standards. State-specific regulations may dictate the scope of practice for nurses engaged in EBP or clinical research, require specific licensure or certification, or outline protocols for patient consent and protection in research studies. By adhering to these requirements, nurses can maintain ethical and legal integrity while promoting the highest standards of care and research ethics.

Understanding the distinctions between EBP and clinical research is vital, and nurses must consult their state board of nursing for specific legislative and licensure requirements. These requirements ensure that nursing practice remains within the bounds of the law, maintains ethical standards, and prioritizes patient safety and well-being in the pursuit of evidence-based care and clinical research.

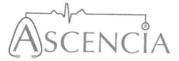

Research Process

The clinical research process is a systematic and structured approach that involves several essential steps, each playing a crucial role in the generation of new knowledge, validation of existing evidence, or exploration of healthcare interventions. These steps guide researchers in conducting rigorous and ethical clinical studies:

- Selecting the topic: The research journey begins with selecting a relevant and meaningful topic. Researchers identify areas where there is a gap in knowledge or where improvements in patient care are needed.

- Finding background information: Before diving into the research, it's crucial to review existing literature and studies related to the chosen topic. This background information helps researchers build a foundation and understand the current state of knowledge.

- Formulating hypotheses: Based on the reviewed literature and the research question, researchers formulate one or more hypotheses. These hypotheses serve as testable statements that the research aims to prove or disprove.

- Designing framework for research: The research design is a critical step that outlines the methodology, data collection methods, and data analysis techniques. Researchers decide whether the study will be observational, experimental, or qualitative, among other considerations.

- Collecting data with approved resources: Researchers collect data according to the research design. This may involve recruiting participants, conducting surveys, performing experiments, or gathering medical records. It's essential to follow ethical guidelines and obtain proper approvals.

- Organizing data: Collected data must be organized systematically for analysis. This includes data entry, coding, and categorization to facilitate meaningful interpretation.

- Evaluating findings: Researchers assess the data to identify patterns, trends, or significant findings. This step involves statistical analyses and other methods to evaluate the research hypothesis.

- Analyzing and interpreting data: Once the data is evaluated, researchers analyze and interpret the results. They determine whether the findings support or refute the hypotheses and draw conclusions.

- Properly citing all sources: Throughout the research process, it is vital to cite all sources of information, including previously published studies, to give credit and provide transparency regarding the sources of evidence.

The clinical research process requires meticulous planning, attention to detail, and adherence to ethical standards. Researchers must also consider factors such as patient consent, data confidentiality, and the use of approved resources. Ultimately, the goal of clinical research is to contribute to the advancement of healthcare knowledge, improve patient outcomes, and inform EBP.

This comprehensive and structured approach to clinical research ensures that studies are conducted rigorously, ethically, and with the highest standards of scientific integrity. It also enables researchers to communicate their findings effectively, allowing for the dissemination of valuable insights to the healthcare community and beyond.

Nursing Teamwork and Collaboration

Delegation and Supervision

Delegation and Supervision Practices

Delegation is one of the core proficiencies of the professional nurse, by which the nurse directs another staff member to fulfill a responsibility or nursing task that they are capable of performing. Effective delegation uses many fundamental nursing skills, such as communication, clinical judgment, time management, and prioritization. The five delegation rights guiding the process encompass the right person, right task, right circumstance, right communication, and right supervision.

The nurse uses clinical judgment to determine whether a task may be delegated to unlicensed assistive personnel (UAP) or another nurse or staff member according to the delegatee's knowledge, education, and experience. The nurse has the responsibility to safeguard the patient, assign the task according to regulations set forth by the state Nurse Practice Act, and follow institutional policies and procedures. The accountability for the task completion lies with the delegating nurse. The patient must be protected from harm.

Because not every circumstance is suitable for delegating, the nurse uses clinical judgment to determine the appropriateness of delegation in each situation. Prior to delegating, the patient's clinical condition and the experience of the delegatee must be assessed. For example, consider the delegation of obtaining vital signs for a newly admitted patient. Assessment of the patient is the responsibility of the nurse. Because the client condition may be unstable, delegation of this task may not be appropriate. However, once the nurse identifies the patient as stable, the routine monitoring of vital signs could be delegated.

Good communication is a crucial aspect of delegation. Determining from the delegatee their familiarity with the task supports the decision to delegate. Furthermore, the delegatee must understand the message conveyed in order to carry out the responsibility. The message must be clearly stated, direct, and concise with sufficient information. The expectation for the task completion must be explicit. When delegating to the nursing assistant the task of obtaining the patient's temperature, comprehensible directions should be provided on how the results are communicated (e.g., inform the delegating nurse and document in the medical record). The receiver of the communication—the nursing assistant in this instance—acknowledges the delegation, asks questions, and provides feedback.

The nurse delegating the responsibility is accountable for the work performed and provides proper supervision, including support, direction, and/or assistance if needed. If the task is not completed by the delegatee, the nurse responsible for the patient care ensures that the duty is fulfilled.

Delegation involves effective time management and prioritization. The nurse must take into consideration the care that is required by the patient and determine the tasks that can be delegated. By

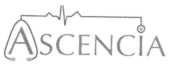

allocating appropriate tasks to another staff member, the nurse gains time to focus on tasks that cannot be delegated and more urgent matters. In this regard, effective delegation allows the nurse to function to the full scope of practice.

Lastly, teamwork is integral to delegation. Nursing staff develop working relationships and trust. Team members have a mutual goal of providing excellent patient care. When the right task is delegated to the right person, positive teamwork can strengthen relationships, improve communication, and create an overall healthy working environment.

Bedside Nurse Supervisory Responsibilities

Amongst the many obligations of the medical-surgical nurse, the role of patient advocate is one that continuously keeps the patient at the forefront of care. The nurse works to protect the patient from harm, maintain patient dignity, coordinate care received, and strive for optimal outcomes. As an ethical duty, the nurse supports the patient by ensuring safe care, assessing the comprehension of decisions, providing education, and identifying the patient's values and preferences.

One aspect of advocacy is supervising the overall care received by the patient. The nurse coordinates and directs care, tracks progress, and develops an understanding of the patient's needs. Because care may be complex, the nurse seeks to ensure that the best quality of care is delivered. For example, when working with unlicensed assistive personnel, the nurse delegates and verifies the completion of tasks. If the patient speaks little English, the nurse coordinates with an interpreter so that the patient has a clear understanding of the care plan. If the patient is subjected to neglectful or abusive behavior, violation of their rights, or any other unethical behavior, the nurse stands by the patient and initiates the chain of command.

As a patient advocate, the nurse supports the principles of patient autonomy and self-determination. The patient has the right to be informed about their medical treatment and choices, and make their own decisions. Often patients consent to family or other caregivers taking part in the decision-making process. The nurse supports the patient and family by bringing forth patient-specific wishes and decisions to the other members of the healthcare team.

Advocacy may be a complex process. Issues like dissent among family members or a declining clinical condition can create a gray area with patient advocacy. Some patients cannot advocate for themselves due to underlying physical and emotional issues. The nurse must communicate well by establishing clear goals with the patient and family and relaying patient preferences to the interprofessional team. More broadly, the nurse must also advocate in local, state, and national forums for the nursing profession (e.g., reducing harm and increasing safe working conditions) because these issues ultimately affect patient care.

Scope of Practice

The nursing scope of practice is defined by the responsibilities that the professional nurse may fulfill under their license. Nursing practice is guided by the standards of practice, the specific state's Nurse Practice Act, codes of ethics, and the institution at which the nurse is employed. The Nurse Practice Act sets the expectations for safe practice, required education, pertinent restrictions, and disciplinary actions. For example, the Nurse Practice Act discusses tasks that may or may not be delegated to unlicensed assistive personnel (UAP), such as activities that require assessment.

The professional nursing role is directed by the standards of care, which define the behaviors of practice and level of competence by which all nurses adhere. The standards are outlined by the state Nurse

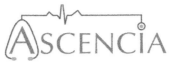

Practice Act and are adopted by professional nursing bodies (e.g., American Nurses Association and Academy of Medical-Surgical Nurses).

The scope of practice is also supported by the policies and procedures of the institution. These policies determine the actions that the nurse may or may not perform in the organization. In many legal situations, the nurse is accountable to the policy. Some states have adopted standardized procedures, in which the Nurse Practice Act specifies that the nurse can perform responsibilities under the institutional standardized procedure that are not typically within the scope of practice. The nurse must have the appropriate training, education, and supervision.

Maintaining one's own competency, skillset, knowledge, and understanding of the nursing scope of practice is the responsibility of the nurse. Because nurses are often delegating and coordinating care, they must also be aware of the scope of practice for other nursing disciplines, such as licensed practical nurse (LPN), licensed vocational nurse (LVN), and unlicensed assistive personnel (nursing assistants). For instance, patient teaching is not a delegable task to a nursing assistant.

Career Development Relationships

Developmental Practices in Nursing

Once the newly licensed nurse enters professional practice, they begin pursuing clinical and professional growth. Orientation is a time devoted to gaining new skills that build upon academic learning and prior professional experience. During the orientation period, the orientee may work with a preceptor, coach, and/or mentor. These relationships allow growth and professional enrichment for both the novice and experienced nurse.

Within a preceptorship, the novice enters a short-term period of working closely with a skilled nurse, referred to as a preceptor. The role of the preceptor is to assess competence and teach skills when a gap is evident. An element of precepting is coaching, although this role may also be distinct. To nurture critical thinking, the novice performs a self-assessment and creates individual goals. The coach may use questions or provide examples that foster reflection. Because the goal is to learn and develop, the coach listens, guides, and provides feedback through the coaching process. In the role of the mentor, the nurse enters a long-term professional relationship with a mentee to enrich professional growth and development. In a supportive environment, the mentee shares difficult encounters, situations, or frustrations. The mentor engages in active listening, provides encouragement, and helps to establish goals.

Comprehending learning theories and learning styles is important for facilitating growth. For example, elements of the adult learning theory state that adults often relate to the purpose of learning, build upon their life experiences, and are internally motivated. A learning style relates to the theory whereby learners gain and comprehend information differently, often through visual aids, hearing spoken words, learning by doing, and writing information or reading words.

The nurse is a lifelong learner. Because the nursing profession encompasses new skills, techniques, and knowledge, the nurse seeks out opportunities for education and growth. Continuing education is required for practice by state boards of nursing, as well as certification. These programs often present knowledge and skills that address practice gaps. In this way, the nurse is accountable to learn current information to provide the best care for the patient.

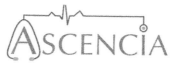

Career development can be found within and outside of the workplace. In the work environment, nurses can serve as charge nurses, preceptors, and mentors, and/or participate in shared governance. Serving on a council at the unit or institutional level encourages nurses to solve problems. Research opportunities and clinical ladders may also be available. Outside of the workplace, professional nursing organizations serve as resources for career development. Participating at the local and/or national level provides opportunities for advocacy, education, and networking on a broader scale. Nurses may also seek specialty certification and higher levels of education.

Nursing Discipline

The discipline of nursing represents a body of knowledge that is continuously growing. Through education, research, and current health issues, new knowledge is built upon the existing theories, frameworks, and standards of practice. The professional nurse must seek to grow in discipline by actively participating in professional engagement, reflective practice, and professional empowerment.

Professional engagement enhances the discipline of nursing because nurses are devoted to the profession and day-to-day work activity. A nurse who is deeply involved and highly committed to patient care is one who brings patient and workflow issues to the forefront, works to resolve problems, and feels empowered to participate at the unit and organizational level. Engaged nurses seek out education, attain certification, and belong to professional organizations. They desire to grow in practice. Active professional engagement leads to a healthier work environment because nurses are involved with decisions and have a voice. As a result, patients have better outcomes and more satisfaction with their care.

Reflective practice is an important part of self-growth for the nurse. The nurse becomes mindful of a situation or perception, further dissects and scrutinizes the thought, and is more open to change as a result. This exercise allows for the nurse to pause and contemplate their actions and attitudes, relations with patients and coworkers, and overall nursing practice. By identifying opportunities for growth and improvement, the nurse can increase their knowledge base and skills or gain a new perspective on their approach.

Reflective practice is also a technique that can be used by the nursing unit. This activity promotes shared decision-making and thoughtful consideration for enhancing patient care, the needs of the nursing unit, and team relations. Reflective practice can lead to improved patient outcomes, improved relations, and professional growth.

The concept of professional empowerment refers to the autonomous and independent practice of the nurse. Making decisions, having a sense of control over one's practice, and believing in oneself are all principles of professional empowerment. With structural empowerment, nurses have access to resources in order to complete their work, which fosters autonomy. Professional empowerment increases job satisfaction among nurses, leads to better quality of care, and aids with retention within the workplace.

Roles and Responsibilities

The nurse must have an understanding of their professional nursing roles and responsibilities in order to practice effectively and keep the patient from harm. The fundamental responsibility of the nurse is to tend to the needs of the patient by initiating the plan of care through the framework of the nursing process. The nurse assesses the patient and collects data, implements the nursing diagnosis, establishes goals, carries out interventions, and evaluates the outcomes. Through the care plan, the nurse guides

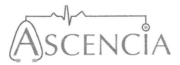

the care of the patient. The role may vary depending upon the type of practice environment, level of education, prior experience, and the skills required.

From knowing roles and responsibilities, the medical-surgical nurse practices to the full scope of their license. Advocating for the patient, understanding preferences and values, and supporting decisions upholds patient autonomy and self-determination. Being familiar with the patient's culture, heritage, and spiritual needs will support the practice of personalized care. Assessing learning needs allows education to be provided in the best manner possible. Seeking out evidence-based practice and nursing research applies current up-to-date knowledge and skills to improve patient outcomes.

The nurse must understand their role because they are accountable to the patient, their institution, and the state board of nursing. Nurses must justify their decisions because they are responsible for the care that they provide. Nursing roles and responsibilities are shaped by the standards of care, the Nursing Code of Ethics, state regulations, professional organizations, and institutional policies and procedures. Developing an understanding of these professional resources will influence the nurse to advocate for the profession and the patients for whom they provide care.

Professional Development

Professional Nursing Practice and Behaviors

The medical-surgical nurse has the duty and responsibility to practice to the best of their ability in order to provide quality care to their patients. As such, maintaining one's own individual set of competencies by seeking out new knowledge, being open to feedback, and growing in practice is a central aspect of nursing. Competencies are a group of abilities needed for the nurse to accomplish their role, established on knowledge, skills, and attitude. The nurse possesses a strong knowledge base, an adept skill set, and high motivation to function competently and autonomously. All nurses perform their duties with a core set of basic competencies, such as application of the nursing process, use of the five medication rights during medication administration, therapeutic communication, and maintaining the dignity of each patient. Within a specialty area, additional competencies are required. For example, the competencies of the medical-surgical nurse include caring for a range of medical and postoperative patients; caring for those at the end-of-life; using technical skills of suctioning, inserting a urinary catheter, and applying a wound dressing; and collaborating with interprofessional team members.

One of the principal responsibilities of the medical-surgical nurse is to coordinate the care the patient receives. Because many caregivers across different healthcare disciplines are involved, collaboration with the interprofessional team has a positive effect on patient outcomes. Caring for the patient is the core objective among the healthcare disciplines, and coordinating the plan together can facilitate the goal. Good communication can profoundly increase care quality and safety. Collaboration can also provide greater breadth of knowledge. For example, reflect on an organizational change to tube feeding products. Bringing all stakeholders together, including the nurse, physician, dietician, pharmacist, and speech and language pathologist, for the review of the new products can streamline patient needs, facilitate communication, and expand knowledge.

Participating in a professional organization is one avenue to advance the nursing profession. Professional organizations broaden the nurse's perspective outside of the work environment and enable collaboration with other nurses who strive to improve nursing practice. Professional organizations support the well-being of the nurse, provide professional development opportunities, encourage

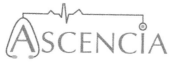

education and certification, advocate for policies and regulations that support the nurse and patient, and advance and disseminate research. Involvement on the local, state, or national level provides the ability to network with nurses, share ideas, gain leadership skills, participate in task forces, attend education courses and conferences, and improve patient care.

Clinical Judgment

Growth in clinical judgment is cultivated over time, shaped by patient experiences, education, advancement of evidence-based practice, and interprofessional collaboration. Clinical judgment pertains to the skill of deducing or making inference about a patient issue or need. A firm knowledge base, personal values, and interactions with the patient contribute to clinical judgment. This knowledge stems from the disease process and patient diagnosis in addition to interactions within the nurse-patient relationship that allow the nurse to perceive the patient's holistic needs. Often patterns in patient care can arise. The experienced nurse can relate issues to previous encounters with prior patients, observations, stories shared by nursing and interprofessional colleagues, and discussions within an educational setting. The many pieces weave together to influence clinical judgment.

When using clinical judgment, the nurse is aware of the patient's problem, interprets the data, and decides how to act. For example, the nurse notices that the patient has shallow breathing with a high respiratory rate and a low-grade fever. The nurse interprets the data, applying the knowledge that the patient recently underwent abdominal surgery. The nurse knows that pain and general anesthesia may affect the patient's breathing pattern, while a low-grade fever is a physiological response following surgery. The nurse makes the clinical judgment that the patient requires a pain relief intervention and increased mobility to improve pain and prevent atelectasis.

Clinical judgment is nurtured through reflective practice. Reflection occurs throughout the clinical judgment process as the patient problem is identified, but also after the event has occurred. The nurse may ask questions, draw inferences, and share their experience with others. As a result, the nurse seeks resources, shares patient encounters, and is receptive to feedback. This process of learning and sharing contributes to the maturation process of clinical judgment.

Peer Review and Educational Needs Assessment

Nursing peer review is a process by which a nurse of the same professional position and clinical expertise evaluates another nurse. After an adverse event occurs related to nursing practice, the nurse responsible for the patient care is evaluated by peers. Considerations are the skill set and stage of practice (e.g., novice or expert nurse), policies in place, education and knowledge required, and confounding factors. The process is intended to be nonpunitive with a recommendation for improvement that may include individual education or policy review, or an organizational practice change. The goal of peer review is to increase accountability and enhance self-regulation of the nursing profession. Nursing peer review is an effective way to support peers, identify areas needing improvement according to nursing practice standards, and ensure the quality of patient care. Some organizations utilize peer evaluation as part of nursing performance evaluations.

An educational (or learning) needs assessment is performed by nurse educators to identify learning needs of the nurse. This process aids in planning nursing education to meet either individual, departmental, or organizational goals. Learning needs can be directly assessed by identifying educational disparities through a gap analysis. Approaches used include providing mock drills and simulation, performing observation, reviewing audits, and keeping abreast of current issues in nursing literature. Other methods include surveys from individual learners, asking for requests, and discussion

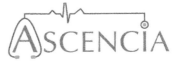

with staff. At the organizational level, safety reports, patient satisfaction surveys, adverse events, risk assessments, and advisory rulings from the state boards of nursing can identify educational needs.

Leadership

Nursing Leadership

Nursing leadership starts at the bedside. As leaders, nurses seek out opportunities for self-growth and inspire others to grow in practice. Nurses impact patient outcomes through actions of advocacy, teaching, motivating, and coordinating care. Nurses can grow in a leadership role by participating in unit-based and hospital-wide councils and joining professional organizations. Undertaking unit responsibilities (including mentor, preceptor, and charge nurse) exemplifies leadership at the bedside.

The charge nurse embodies leadership by representing the nursing staff team during a shift. Coordinating the unit flow, the charge nurse tracks patient discharges and assigns new admissions. The charge nurse is aware of the competence of each team member to assign and delegate the proper tasks. They respond to patient emergencies, provide customer service, and advocate for the bedside nurse. If supplies are needed, the charge nurse works to obtain equipment for nurses to perform in their care. Furthermore, the charge nurse is knowledgeable of organizational policies and procedures to serve as a resource and direct care.

The nursing staff serve under the nurse manager, who represents the leader of the unit. The nurse manager is part of the nursing administration team, reporting to a director of nursing (DON) or chief nursing officer (CNO). Ensuring that the nursing unit is functioning well on a day-to-day basis, the nurse manager hires new staff and is responsible for nursing schedules. The nurse manager verifies that the unit activity is working according to organizational goals and procedures. They maintain the unit finances, address safety issues and problems, and discipline staff when needed.

Regulatory and Compliance Standards

Administrative nurse leaders are nurse managers, clinical practice leaders, and others who preside over a nursing unit or clinical setting. Serving as a liaison between the organization and the frontline nurse, the administrative nurse leader supports the clinical nurse in their role to provide quality patient care, while also instilling organizational goals and values. The nurse leader ensures that frontline nurses meet the needs of the patient and provide an environment in which nurses can competently deliver care. Among responsibilities to support clinical care, nurse leaders instill a vision for the nursing unit, oversee daily operations, identify staff needs, support evidence-based practice, provide resources, advance patient care initiatives, and advocate for the nursing profession.

In the administrative nursing role, nurse leaders adhere to leadership regulatory and compliance standards, which are defined by professional nursing bodies. The nurse maintains a registered nurse license, possesses strong patient care experience, practices within the state board of nursing scope of practice, and frequently holds a higher academic degree. For example, nurse managers often hold at least a bachelor of science in nursing (BSN). Administrative nurse leaders frequently maintain a leadership certification. Furthermore, they have clinical expertise, as well as a comprehensive understanding of quality healthcare described by accreditation and regulatory agencies. Nurse leaders embody professional qualities, like emotional intelligence, enthusiasm, honesty, and transparency.

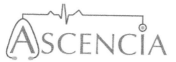

The nurse leader builds a diverse team and fosters growth among nursing staff. They evaluate staff competence and are accountable for ensuring that the staff have appropriate education, licenses, and certification to meet their job description and practice according to nursing standards and institutional policies. Strong communication skills allow for effective communication among stakeholders of the nursing unit (e.g., patients, nursing staff, and interdisciplinary colleagues). When conflicts arise, the nurse leader meets with those involved to determine a resolution or course of action. The development of employees is supported by the nurse leader through constructive feedback, encouragement of lifelong learning, and appropriate delegation.

Within the healthcare environment, administrative nurse leaders are responsible for the business operation of the nursing unit. They hire new staff and oversee scheduling to determine a sufficient amount of personnel for patient care. Among other business skills, the nurse leader performs cost-benefit analyses, oversees the unit finances, and utilizes accounting skills. As a systems thinker, they are able to see the nursing unit as a larger part of the organization and work towards strategic goals. As agents of change, the administrative nurse leader welcomes new ideas and information. The nurse leader instills a vision that enables others to act towards a common goal.

Organizational Structure

The organizational structure provides a hierarchy for decision-making within the nursing department. By illustrating the reporting authority, the organizational structure delineates roles and differentiates responsibilities. It dictates the way information flows to accomplish strategic goals. A chain of command is established so that patient safety issues may be escalated for a resolution.

In a standard organization, the chief nursing officer (CNO) is the executive nurse leader at the top of the organizational structure. The role is involved with strategic and business planning for the organization. The CNO supports the nursing unit management, oversees the financial budget, establishes nursing standards of practice, directs nursing education needs, sets forth new policies and guidelines, and supports best practice. Associate chief nursing officers (ACNO) may serve under the CNO as executive nurse leaders and participate in nursing strategic planning.

The director of nursing (DON) reports to the CNO. The DON may oversee several nursing units or clinical areas, such as a number of medical-surgical units. Reporting to the DON, nurse managers are responsible for one nursing unit and are closest in the organizational structure to the frontline nursing staff. They oversee the daily operations of the nursing unit.

The direct care nursing staff report to the nurse manager, including the charge nurse, registered nurse (RN), licensed practical nurse (LPN)/ licensed vocational nurse (LVN), and unlicensed assistive personnel (UAP) (i.e., nursing assistants). The charge nurse is responsible for the staff who provide bedside care during the shift. They may make decisions in the absence of the nurse manager, direct and coordinate workflow, and act as a resource. Charge nurses may or may not be assigned direct patient care.

The RN, LPN/ LVN, and UAP have an indirect hierarchy, although all positions report to the nurse manager. The RN holds more education than an LPN/LVN and practices in a broader scope. For example, the RN can assess patients, delegate to others, administer medication, and have greater autonomy. In some organizations, the RN is responsible for guiding the LPN/ LVN. The LPN/ LVN scope is more restrictive and these nurses usually provide a more basic level of patient care. UAPs assist the patient with activities of daily living, such as hygiene, feeding, toileting, and ambulating. Their care is directed by the LPN/ LVN or RN.

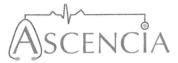

When working for an institution, the nurse is familiar with facility-specific terminology and organizational structure. Nurses are accountable for their care delivery. They must be aware of policies and procedures, the chain of command, and other facility-specific operations to provide safe quality care. For example, one facility may use yellow as a fall precaution color to align with the national color system. However, other agencies may not have adopted the same color scheme and use orange. Knowing these variations is important in protecting patients from harm.

Nursing Philosophy

A nursing philosophy is a set of intrinsic values by which a nurse practices. A philosophy is molded by life values, an academic foundation, personal experiences, and beliefs about nursing professional practice. For example, a nurse who is attracted to the profession because she cared for her sick family member has a distinct outlook on nursing because of this deep personal experience. Common themes may relate to caring, human dignity, ethics, quality of care, and professionalism. A nursing philosophy gives the nurse purpose that creates the impetus, motivation, and willingness to practice. When a nurse practices according to their own philosophy, their values are reflected in their work.

Nurse leaders often develop skills and practice according to a nursing leadership philosophy. The philosophy clarifies the manner in which the nurse leader is driven, according to their values, personal convictions about nursing, and expectations. Philosophy statements give insight into leadership skills, leadership styles, and the way in which the nurse leader interacts with staff. These values guide decision-making, actions, and work ethic. The nurse leader's philosophy influences the nursing unit goals and sets the tone for the work environment. A leader who lives by their philosophy and embodies these principles through words and actions is the essence of authentic leadership. An authentic leader is rooted in their core beliefs and guided by their philosophy. They exemplify their own values, and this builds trust in their staff, improves patient outcomes, and encourages a healthy work environment.

Leadership Models

Leadership styles are sets of characteristics or traits that a leader uses to manage their team. As a result, leadership styles can profoundly affect the nursing unit environment, staff relationships, quality of care, and the overall operations. Among the different types of leadership styles are autocratic, democratic, servant, transformational, laissez-faire, transactional, and situational. Some styles may be more appropriate than others, depending on the situation at hand.

With autocratic leadership, the nurse leader makes decisions without any staff participation. Often this type of leader is very effective with delegating tasks and managing emergencies. If the leader does not communicate enough information, staff may feel disempowered. Democratic leadership, on the other hand, is more collaborative. Staff input is a factor in decisions. Because the leader is effective with building relationships, the work environment is positive. Often there is a goal of improving the system without placing blame. However, decision-making may not be instantaneous if participation is encouraged among all staff. The leader may not be efficient in making independent decisions as well. The servant leader is focused on meeting individual needs and developing the employee. They are inclusive, empathetic, and focus on maximizing strengths. However, decisions may not be timely, the team may develop a dependency on the leader, and the leader may lack authority.

Transformational leaders work towards a greater vision of nursing within the organization. They inspire employees to achieve goals. The strengths of a transformational leader include employee job satisfaction, high quality patient outcomes, and providing quality mentoring. Drawbacks may include lack of clear guidelines, insufficient structure, and leader job burnout. Laissez-faire leadership occurs

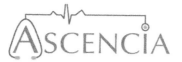

when the nurse leader avoids a situation, neglects to provide feedback, and offers little supervision. If the team is highly experienced or motivated, laissez-faire may be a useful leadership style to empower independent decision-making among staff. However, this type of style is often associated with a negative work environment and poor job satisfaction.

The transactional leader is concerned with productivity and performance. They operate by managing tasks and expecting compliance with policies and procedures. Tactics used are rewards and punishment. This leadership style may decrease errors but does not promote job satisfaction. With situational leadership, the nurse leader adapts to the needs of the nurse or the organization. But because the situational nurse leader is so flexible, the organizational goals may not be efficiently met.

Nursing Care Delivery Systems

A nursing care delivery model provides a systematic framework for nurses to deliver care to patients. The purpose of the delivery model is to organize care in a way that efficiently allocates resources, serves patient needs, meets healthcare system goals, optimizes nursing staff, and supports nursing autonomy. Models vary among institutions. They are influenced by many components, such as the nurse's responsibilities, distribution of tasks, economic factors, patient and nurse satisfaction, the means to collaborate among the interprofessional team, and nurse management. In this way, the delivery model is one factor that sets the tone of the work environment. Because delivery of care may be complex, models support the ability for the nurse to effectively communicate, make decisions, coordinate care, and provide for their patient's needs to facilitate high-quality patient outcomes. Examples of nursing care delivery models include total patient care, primary care nursing, functional nursing, and team nursing.

The total patient care delivery model allows nurses to work one-on-one with an assigned group of patients. The assignments are considered on a shift-by-shift basis by the charge nurse. In this regard, continuity is less prioritized than the primary care nursing model described below. During the shift, the nurse would assume total care to meet the complete needs of the patient. An individual working relationship is established with the patient, unlike that of team nursing. If LPNs/LVNs or UAPs are present, an RN would oversee and delegate the care. An advantage of this model is nursing independence over the care that they provide. Shortcomings of total patient care include that assignments may change with different shifts. The patient may be cared for by multiple nurses throughout their stay and nobody is coordinating the overall care.

With primary care nursing, the main focus of the model is continuity of care, which means the same nurse cares for the patient during their stay. One nurse is assigned to manage the patient care from admission through discharge and guides the care plan even when they are not on location. In the primary nurse's absence, the care would be delegated to another nurse according to the plan determined by the primary nurse. The primary nurse is responsible and accountable for care delivery. Different skill levels may be used, such as a novice or an expert nurse. However, in a nontraditional clinical area, this model is not successful when nurses have a variety of responsibilities and limited presence with the patient.

The functional nursing care delivery model refers to the assignment of tasks by a charge nurse. The charge nurse takes into consideration the knowledge and skills required for the patient's care. This model is beneficial when the skill set of the team is varied. Novice nurses can be assigned more basic tasks than expert nurses. The task-oriented nature of this model necessitates the dependency upon protocols and policies by the charge nurse. Weaknesses include that the model of care is so task-focused that it may not support nursing autonomy, professional development, or holistic care of the patient.

Nursing Teamwork and Collaboration

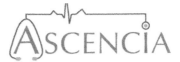

Often there is little regard to differentiation of the distinct nursing roles or academic preparation (i.e., RN, LPN). There is also a lack of clear accountability for the care provided. Often, the charge nurse or nurse manager is responsible for delegating tasks and communicating patient reports.

In team nursing, a team of nurses delivers patient care instead of one individual nurse. The nurses work collaboratively together with a shared collective responsibility to provide care. Because the combined team holds diverse skill sets, educational backgrounds, and distinct experiences, they provide a range of expertise to serve the needs of the patient. A registered nurse performs as the team leader, who is accountable for the care provided. This role requires leadership skills and good communication. The team nursing model may be beneficial for newer and more novice staff, and it can provide the opportunity for mentoring if the nursing unit does not contain many highly skilled staff. Additionally, this type of care delivery model often leads to a supportive environment, better communication among staff, and improved patient outcomes. Yet, a drawback is that nurses may have poor job satisfaction if communication about each nurse's function is not clearly defined. Furthermore, the same team may not work together on every shift.

Change Management

Because healthcare is frequently transforming, the administrative nurse has a responsibility to facilitate this process. Different change theories exist to achieve success and guide the nurse leader. Essential components of change management are successful planning and coordination, communication of new changes, and staff support. One example of a change theory is ADKAR, an acronym for Awareness, Desire, Knowledge, Ability, and Reinforcement. The first step is to create awareness among the staff that there is a desire to change. The nursing staff gains understanding of the purpose, asks questions, and provides feedback. Next, there is a desire among the staff to want to change. Employees may be tentative; in which case the nurse leader offers encouragement. Third, knowledge is delivered through means of education, in-services, and sharing of resources. Fourth, the ability to change is demonstrated through pilot trials, when the opportunity for adjustments can be addressed. Finally, reinforcement of the change is provided through follow up and feedback so that staff do not return to former processes.

Recruitment and Retention

One of the goals of the administrative nurse is to recruit and retain nursing staff to effectively provide high-quality patient care. Many variables in the work environment occur, such as the amount of resources available, the complexity of care and skills required, the staffing of the nursing unit (including turnover and staff vacancies), and the organizational strategic plan. The nurse manager collaborates with the human resources department to recruit a diverse and talented nursing staff. The nurse leader is responsible for interviewing selected candidates and hiring the recruited nurses.

Staff recruitment and retention requires striking a balance between organizational goals and nursing job role satisfaction. The administrative nurse has an important responsibility of retaining nurses that are hired. Not only does nursing turnover affect an organization financially, but it also can impact productivity, morale, and patient outcomes. High turnover can lead to medical error and decreased patient satisfaction. Nurses are influenced by recognition of the care that they provide, their day-to-day workload, competitive wages, available resources, opportunities of growth, and financial benefits (e.g., tuition reimbursement).

The novice nurse is vulnerable to turnover due to their lack of confidence in the professional role, as well as insufficient support. Providing the novice nurse with resources upon hire can make them feel valued from the beginning of their employment. An in-depth orientation with a skilled preceptor can

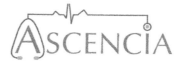

improve retention. The nurse manager promotes preceptor education and encourages time for the preceptor to teach during the shift. The administrative nurse can also support the novice nurse by facilitating access to resources such as residency programs, newly licensed nurse support groups, and mentoring.

Beyond orientation, the administrative nurse has the responsibility to retain the nursing staff as the nurse grows in the professional role. When nurses are satisfied and happy with their jobs, they are less apt to vacate their position. Nurses appreciate feeling valued by their nurse leader. For example, the nurse who is recognized for performance feels a high level of appreciation by their manager. Other examples include role autonomy, competitive wages, paid time off, scheduling flexibility, compensation for education and nursing conferences, and a manageable workload.

Retention is impacted by leader competence, as well as a healthy work environment. Staff members value a nurse leader who appears adept at their role. The administrative nurse can invest in their own leadership growth, be a role model, and practice according to their philosophy. Applying evidence-based elements of a healthy work environment can positively increase the nursing unit atmosphere. High-functioning work environments are characterized by effective communication, transparency, staff engagement, strong team relationships, a shared vision of the nursing unit, and celebrations of successes.

Employee Engagement

Staff engagement is key to a healthy work environment. When nurses lack enthusiasm, experience burnout, and exhibit poor morale, job performance and patient outcomes can be negatively affected. However, when nurses are invested in their position, feel connected to the organization, and have a positive attitude, they often provide a higher quality of care. Job engagement can help nurses feel motivated, dedicated to their responsibilities, and self-directed. As a result, nurses are less apt to vacate their positions, and patient satisfaction improves.

Nurse managers, educators, and executive leaders play a pivotal role in creating a positive work environment where nurses can feel invested in the organization. Career development—such as education, certification, and participation in a clinical ladder—can be supported through reimbursement, flexible scheduling, and incentives. Staff participation in the charge nurse, preceptor, or mentor roles provide nurses an opportunity to serve as leaders, resources, and teachers. With shared governance, nurses participate in decision-making at the unit or organizational level, leading to empowerment. Continuing education and attendance at conferences and symposiums allow nurses to seek new knowledge.

Adopting innovative ideas and evidence-based practices motivates nursing staff to work towards a goal. Some nursing units organize journal clubs led by clinical nurses that review literature and incorporate best practices. For example, an organizational goal could be decreasing hospital-acquired conditions. A nurse manager informs the nursing staff that the unit has increased hospital-acquired pressure injuries, one of their quality indicators. The journal club appraises the literature and decides to implement the practice of two RNs assessing patient skin on admission to verify the patient's skin condition. Through shared decision-making, the nurses plan the initiative and motivate other nursing staff to improve outcomes. This process leads to staff empowerment, a shared vision among the unit, and motivation to accomplish the goal.

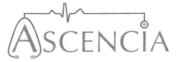

Staff Advocacy

When challenging situations arise on the nursing unit, the administrative nurse can serve as an advocate for the healthcare team. Stressful events can impact job performance and care delivery. Examples include an organizational change, conflict, patient death, chaos, unplanned event, crisis, and sentinel event. The nurse leader creates a supportive environment to help nurses feel valued. Positive attributes during strenuous circumstances include listening, being objective and calm, debriefing, offering compassion and empathy, and maintaining a non-punitive position. If the situation involves one individual nurse, the nurse leader may support a break or relief from patient care or a different patient assignment.

Conflict Management

Conflict is a circumstance that can arise within any team and is often considered unavoidable. Although conflict is difficult, positive change and resolution can be a successful outcome when managed properly. Types of conflict identified in nursing include struggles among nursing staff, interprofessional colleagues, patients and families, and leadership. Complex situations may arise due to staff perceptions, emotions, or assumptions. As a result, communication breakdowns, poor collegial relations, and stressful conditions ensue. Effective conflict management is a skill acquired by the nurse manager, so the team works well together to deliver patient care. Conflict management encompasses collaboration, effective communication, and teamwork, which reflect a healthy work environment.

The administrative nurse aims to achieve a resolution among the parties involved and uses strategies to address conflict. Different theories on conflict management styles exist (e.g., Thomas Kilmann Conflict Model) and often the situation determines the style and communication used. For example, the nurse leader may use compromise to resolve a conflict. Addressing conflict as early as possible avoids an escalation of the situation. Listening to both parties calmly and in a nonjudgmental manner provides an opportunity for everyone to express a viewpoint and feel valued. Clarifying the issues helps to identify a goal and move towards resolution. The nurse leader seeks a workable solution for both people. Furthermore, nurse managers empower staff by coaching successful conflict management strategies.

Financial Stewardship

Financial stewardship is a thoughtful approach to managing resources and eliminating unnecessary costs, while considering the quality of care required by the patient. Nursing leaders work within a budget to successfully manage resources, including nursing staff, supplies, and equipment. Costs for the nursing staff include productive working hours providing direct care, as well as nonproductive hours (e.g., for education, training, and paid time off). The operating budget factors in non-salary costs (e.g., patient supplies, equipment, and office supplies), which is affected by patient volume. A separate capital budget relates to the organizational strategic goals, such as purchasing a costly item for a clinical area.

Clinical nurses at the bedside are also financial stewards. Nurses can be mindful of fiscal responsibility by working within scheduled hours and not creating the need for overtime. As a charge nurse, appropriate staffing of the unit eliminates the need for extra staff. Thoughtful utilization of supplies reduces waste. For example, nurses can determine the number of supplies (e.g., products or linen) needed prior to care, without bringing extra items to the bedside.

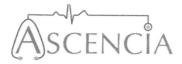

Disaster Planning and Management

Healthcare organizations define emergency preparedness and response procedures for when disasters occur. Disasters strike unexpectedly, and vary depending on the event location and nature of the circumstance. Disasters occur within the healthcare facility or in the community due to a man-made or natural occurrence. Internal disasters include fire, hazardous material (hazmat) incidents, radiation spills, active shooters, and high census. External disasters (e.g., hurricanes, accidents, flooding, wildfires, or infectious disease) frequently impact the surrounding community, and often affect the healthcare facility. Daily organizational operations and normal patient care routines are often disrupted. The nursing staff must be ready to receive information from the organizational leadership, promptly respond, and adapt to changing needs.

The Emergency Operations Plan (EOP) describes the plan and structure for the organization's emergency response to all hazards. The plan contents may include the instructions for plan implementation, staff notification, bed availability, surge capacity, staffing information, and debriefing. For example, mass casualty incidents (MCIs) lead to a large number of patients, which may be more than the healthcare facility can accommodate. Natural disasters may require the healthcare facility to secure the safety of their own site. The main purpose of the EOP is to ensure that patients will be cared for effectively with minimal disruption. The plan must be organized in order to respond to a worst-case scenario and avoid chaos. Tasks must be delegated and the flow of information determined, often through an incident command structure.

Patients admitted on a large-scale may have traumatic injuries and immediate needs. As a result, capacity will need to be increased. By discharging those who are stable, reallocating physical space, and staffing additional personnel, more patient care can be delivered. The triaging of patients is fulfilled according to a classification system. The non-urgent patient does not need immediate attention (e.g., those with a minor laceration or closed fracture). An urgent patient requires treatment and may have sustained injuries that are not life-threatening (e.g., open fractures or large wounds). The emergent patient has the highest priority with life-threatening injuries and needs immediate attention (e.g., trauma, amputations, or severe respiratory distress).

In order to most effectively respond, the hospital typically uses four phases of disaster management (mitigation, preparedness, response, and recovery). During the mitigation phase, the goal is to reduce harm as much as possible. The community risks are broadly assessed before disaster occurs and resources are identified at that time. The preparedness phase is the creation and activation of the emergency plan. The plan details are determined by the care and needs required by the victims; establishment of responsibilities; and identification of resources, supplies, and provisions. Training and mock drills identify gaps that need to be addressed. The third phase, response, is initiated once the emergency occurs in an effort to save lives and prevent further damage. Finally, recovery is a return to a stable state, while addressing psychological and emotional needs and providing ongoing support.

The hospital incident command system (HICS) manages the disaster response. The framework is adapted from the National Incident Management System established by the Federal Emergency Management Act (FEMA). The HCIS outlines the organizational response in a streamlined and concise manner. Elements consist of establishing goals, identifying needs, creating a plan, utilizing the various positions within the hospital, providing support, and communicating instructions. A designated centralized location is identified as the hospital command center, where much of the communication will occur. Within an established hierarchy, the command center accepts the disaster, as well as oversees the response and

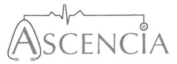

resolution. Responsibilities are distributed as needed, and the number of people involved with the HCIS is flexible, depending on the disaster situation. For example, a smaller emergency within the hospital would require fewer staff members than a larger, external one.

At the top of the hierarchy of the HCIS, an incident commander serves as the overall leader. Within the incident command team, other roles may be included. For example, a security and safety officer will communicate with local law enforcement to ensure the safety of the hospital staff and patients. A liaison officer is responsible for speaking with external organizations and emergency response partners about the hospital's bed availability and overall status. A public information officer coordinates communications, such as an internal hotline or approved announcements to the media. The four main branches that fall under incident command include operations, planning, logistics, and finance. Leaders are assigned to these subdivisions and each team is designated with their own responsibilities and objectives. The operations team manages all the hospital operations, including infrastructure, security, hazmat, clinical units, information technology, and social services. The patient care division (within the operations team) is led by a medical director, with additional leaders for critical care, medical-surgical units, respiratory therapists, pharmacists, and others. The planning team will coordinate the plan documentation and dissemination of information. The logistics team will direct the resources, equipment, supplies, and workers. Finally, the finance team will oversee expenses and payments. A goal for the HCIS framework is collaboration, effective communication, minimized chaos, and successful management of the disaster.

Practice Test #1

1. The nurse is caring for a 94-year-old patient admitted with lower abdominal pain. The patient reports that she has not voided since yesterday. Her bladder scan shows 1200 mL of urine in the bladder and an order for an indwelling urinary catheter was obtained. The nurse knows that she should follow the new CAUTI bundle to reduce the risk of a hospital-acquired urinary tract infection. Which element is included?
   a. Maintaining the urine collection bag on an IV pole so that the tubing is free from kinks.
   b. Cleansing the catheter insertion site daily with a hospital-grade disinfecting wipe.
   c. Assessing the clinical indication for the indwelling catheter daily.
   d. Changing the urine collection bag q72h to prevent the harboring of bacteria.

2. The nurse is working with a nursing assistant and caring for four patients in her assignment. They each have complex problems. Their conditions have been assessed by the nurse already this shift. Which task is LEAST appropriate to delegate to a nursing assistant?
   a. Providing a complete bath to an 81-year-old patient admitted yesterday for a full-thickness sacral pressure injury
   b. Feeding lunch to a newly admitted 90-year-old patient diagnosed with dysphagia as a result of a stroke
   c. Assisting a 75-year-old patient who had a right hip replacement three days ago into the chair
   d. Ambulating a cooperative and disoriented 83-year-old patient admitted last night in the hallway

3. What is the expected effect of injury or fever on caloric needs?
   a. Metabolic demand causes caloric needs to increase
   b. Homeostasis reduces metabolic demand and caloric needs remain the same
   c. Caloric needs will decrease as metabolic demand increases
   d. Insulin production lowers to provide increased glucose availability

4. Which of the following is NOT a key aspect of physical and environmental workplace safety in nursing practice?
   a. Proper disposal of biohazardous materials
   b. Regular maintenance of medical equipment
   c. Proper hand hygiene protocols
   d. Adequate nurse-to-patient ratios

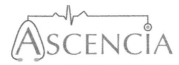

5. The nurse is administering a patient's medications. She identifies the patient and performs the medication pass according to the five medication rights. As she is finishing, the patient states, "I am having pain. Could you please bring me pain medication?" The nurse leaves the patient bedside, obtains the medication, returns to the patient room, and reopens the patient medication administration record. Before handing the medication to the patient, the nurse performs which of next steps in the medication administration process?

    a.   She scans the patient identification bracelet with the barcode scanner, then scans the medication barcode.

    b.   She opens the medication package, then places the tablet into a medication cup.

    c.   She asks the patient for his name and date of birth, then scans the bracelet with the barcode scanner.

    d.   She asks the patient for his name and date of birth, then verifies the identification with the medication administration record.

6. How is it determined that an intervention met the previously set goals and outcomes?

    a.   Data, observation, and feedback are used.

    b.   The patient states they feel better.

    c.   The provider states the disease process is improved.

    d.   Some of the outcomes are met.

7. What is the main goal of performance improvement projects that are aimed at improving documentation?

    a.   To reduce occurrences of double orders

    b.   To diminish communication among interdisciplinary teams

    c.   To decrease speed of information delivery

    d.   To duplicate claim capture

8. A 26-year-old male patient is admitted for an appendectomy. When his surgery is completed, he is transferred to the post-anesthesia care unit (PACU). The PACU nurse assumes care of the patient and knows that the early phase of recovery (PACU phase 1) means that:

    a.   Anesthesia recovery and restoration of baseline vital signs are the goal.

    b.   Pain must be managed effectively so that the patient can transition to home.

    c.   Patients who are intubated need to be monitored for extubation.

    d.   The nurse assesses the patient's swallowing ability with a monitored sip test.

9. A 69-year-old female patient is readmitted after receiving treatment with ampicillin-sulbactam for a diabetic wound infection. She is now reporting abdominal cramping, nausea, and frequent diarrhea. What is the nurse's FIRST priority in providing care?

    a.   Send a stool specimen to the lab.

    b.   Document ampicillin-sulbactam as an allergy.

    c.   Initiate contact precautions.

    d.   Notify the doctor.

10. A nurse is teaching a patient with acute kidney failure ways to improve kidney function. Which of the following statements indicates patient understanding?

    a.   "I should eat a diet high in protein."

    b.   "I will need to be scheduled to get a fistula for dialysis."

    c.   "I will limit my sodium intake to less than 2000 milligrams per day."

    d.   "I can eat all of the oranges I want since they are lower calorie and healthy."

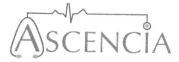

11. The licensed nurse delegates the task of calculating oral intake and output (I&O) to the nursing assistant for a patient who underwent a laparoscopic cholecystectomy. As part of the five rights of delegation, the nurse logs into the electronic medical record and confirms that the nursing assistant completed the task. Which of the following delegation rights does this most pertain to?
   a. The right task
   b. The right circumstance
   c. The right communication
   d. The right supervision

12. The medical-surgical nurse has responded to a call light, and the patient has stated that he is having stabbing chest pain rated as 8/10. The patient has a recent cardiac history, with cardiac stents placed post-myocardial infarction 2 months ago. What type of assessment should the nurse perform on this patient?
   a. Comprehensive
   b. Focused
   c. Behavioral
   d. Head-to-toe

13. The medical-surgical nurse is caring for a patient who has had a recent weight loss of over 15 kilograms through binging and purging with laxatives and has been admitted for weakness and a syncopal episode. The nurse reviews the patient's most recent assessment and vital signs. Which of the following findings should be reported to the healthcare provider immediately?
   a. Hair loss
   b. Overactive bowel sounds
   c. Irregular, thready pulse with a rate of 110 bpm
   d. Last period four months ago

14. A 45-year-old man is admitted to the nursing unit for pneumonia. His initial assessment showed a temperature of 101.5 °F/38.6 °C and a respiratory rate of 24 breaths per minute. His lung sounds have rhonchi, and he has copious amounts of yellow/green sputum with a productive cough. Now three days into his hospital stay, the current assessment indicates a temperature of 99.8 °F/37.6 °C, respiratory rate of 19 breaths per minute, clear lung sounds, and pale-yellow sputum production. The nurse sees that he is scheduled for ceftriaxone 1 gm IV during the shift. Which action BEST supports antimicrobial stewardship by the nurse?
   a. Talking with the medical provider regarding the appropriate medication route
   b. Continuing the administration of the antibiotic as ordered
   c. Obtaining a sputum culture to confirm that the patient still has pneumonia
   d. Asking the patient for his medication allergies.

15. What stage of the nursing process will be revisited if it is found that an intervention is not effective?
   a. Diagnosis
   b. Assessment
   c. Intervention
   d. Evaluation

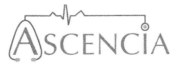

16. The registered nurse is caring for an 84-year-old female patient admitted for aspiration pneumonia. She would like to delegate the task of administering an antibiotic through IV push to a licensed practical nurse (LPN). She is unsure if this task is within the responsibilities that the LPN may fulfill. In which location is she most likely able to confirm this action?
   a.   A resource on the nursing scope of practice published by her professional nursing organization
   b.   A nursing textbook that provides an in-depth overview of current nursing issues
   c.   A website on the Board of Nursing that describes the LPN scope of practice
   d.   A medication insert pamphlet for the antibiotic to be administered

17. The nurse is placing ECG leads on a patient after the provider orders telemetry monitoring. What is the best method to ensure that the electrodes are placed for optimal reading?
   a.   Affix electrodes per order or facility policy
   b.   Apply lotion to areas to prevent irritation
   c.   Place over hair and press down firmly to ensure contact
   d.   Remove when patient is moving around too much

18. The hospital system has activated the emergency response plan. The medical-surgical nurse expects that a large number of patients will be admitted in response to a flooding disaster in the community. The nurse can best prepare to admit new patients by:
   a.   participating in mock drills to identify gaps in the emergency plan.
   b.   identifying resources so that the victims' psychological and emotional needs can be supported.
   c.   assessing the flood risks by knowing the evacuation route.
   d.   attending discharge planning rounds with the healthcare team.

19. Which organization is responsible for accrediting healthcare facilities and ensuring they adhere to rigorous safety and quality standards?
   a.   American Nurses Association (ANA)
   b.   State Board of Nursing
   c.   Centers for Medicare & Medicaid Services (CMS)
   d.   The Joint Commission

20. An 80-year-old male patient is admitted to the nursing unit. He is disheveled and appears emaciated. The clothes he is wearing are malodorous and stained with urine. His dentures and glasses are missing. Upon assessment, the nurse notes that he is only oriented to self and place. There is partial-thickness skin loss to his elbows and sacrum. The patient is also deconditioned and has difficulty ambulating. He reports not seeing his son recently. What should be the nurse's FIRST intervention provided?
   a.   Report the situation immediately to the facility abuse officer.
   b.   Notify the social worker to consult with the patient.
   c.   Call the patient's son and notify him of his father's admission.
   d.   Treat the pressure injuries per MD order or facility protocol.

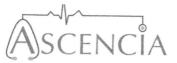

21. The nurse is admitting a 52-year-old male patient to the nursing unit for severe abdominal pain. He is in a side-lying position with guarding and reports nausea, a low-grade fever, and right lower quadrant pain at home. How can the nurse most effectively communicate the task of vital signs when delegating to the nursing assistant?

   a. "Could you please obtain the vital signs as quickly as possible and report the results directly to me."
   b. "Could you please take a set of vital signs when you are performing your rounds and document the results in the medical record."
   c. "Could you please help the patient into the bathroom, take a set of vital signs, and write the results on a slip of paper for me."
   d. The nurse does not delegate the task of vital signs for this patient.

22. A 78-year-old male is admitted for an open reduction and internal fixation (ORIF) after sustaining a fall on ice and fracturing his left hip. The medical-surgical nurse provides a handoff to the perioperative nurse before the patient is transferred to the operating room. What is an accurate statement about the actions that take place before the incision is made?

   a. The pre-procedure verification is completed once the patient is given anesthesia.
   b. The timeout is conducted with the surgical team that will be present once the surgery is complete.
   c. The perioperative nurse initiates the preoperative checklist to ensure documentation is present.
   d. The surgical team jointly agrees upon the patient identification, surgical site, and procedure.

23. The nurse has assessed a patient and obtained vital signs. An unlicensed assistive personnel alerts the nurse that another patient has developed shortness of breath. After stabilizing the second patient, the nurse finishes charting the first patient. When should the assessment be timed for on the electronic health record?

   a. Current time of charting
   b. At the start of the shift
   c. At the time the assessment occurred
   d. At the hour of assessment

24. What is one of the key steps involved in service recovery in healthcare that reinforces the commitment to patient-centered care?

   a. Recognition of the issue and immediate corrective actions
   b. Continuous monitoring of the situation and implementation of preventive measures
   c. Identifying the problem and assigning blame
   d. Delays in addressing patient concerns to prioritize administrative processes

25. What is a main goal of utilizing alternative communication formats for sensory impairments?

   a. To reduce the need for face-to-face communication
   b. To improve health literacy in modalities understandable to the patient
   c. To assign a representative to make decisions for patients with sensory deficits
   d. To eliminate the need for translation services

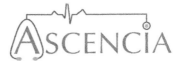

26. During the bedside shift report, the oncoming nurse disagrees with how the outgoing nurse cared for the patient during his shift. He exclaims, "You always leave patients for me this way!" The nurse manager walks by and hears the exchange. She knows that the best way to manage the conflict is to meet with the two nurses and:
   a. consider ideas for how the issue can be remedied.
   b. express her concern about the negative communication.
   c. listen to both sides of the story so that she can clarify the issue.
   d. ask the outgoing nurse to provide his care according to the hospital policy.

27. A nurse is caring for a 56-year-old male patient who reports arthritic pain with a verbal pain score of 8/10. The patient has PRN orders for oxycodone 2.5 mg, but the tablet is available as 5 mg. The nurse asks her coworker to waste half of the tablet by the medication-dispensing cabinet, and her coworker correctly observes the nurse dispose of the waste in which of the following receptacles?
   a. Regulated medical waste
   b. Controlled substance waste
   c. Sharps container
   d. Sink

28. The nurse is assessing a patient's pain. The patient describes it as stabbing. What category of patient data is this considered?
   a. Objective
   b. Personal
   c. Subjective
   d. Quantitative

29. A nurse listens as a patient tells their medical history and personal concerns. The nurse holds the patient's hand and states an understanding of the feelings that the patient is expressing. What is this concept called?
   a. Empathy
   b. Implicit bias
   c. Sympathy
   d. Active listening

30. A nurse manager is investigating a new nursing care delivery model that would better serve the needs of the nursing unit. She wants to organize care more efficiently and optimize the skills of the nursing staff. The unit has many novice nurses and the nurse manager would like to enhance their skill sets and provide them with an opportunity for mentoring. Furthermore, she feels that the experienced nurses could develop leadership skills. Which type of nursing care delivery model should she most consider?
   a. Total patient care
   b. Primary care
   c. Functional nursing
   d. Team nursing

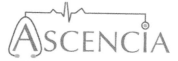

31. Why are Nursing-Sensitive Indicators (NSIs), such as adverse events and staffing models, important for evolving nursing practice models?
   a. NSIs primarily focus on cost-saving measures in healthcare.
   b. NSIs help healthcare organizations prioritize marketing strategies.
   c. NSIs provide insights into the quality of nursing care and its impact on patient outcomes.
   d. NSIs are useful for identifying new medical treatments.

32. Who is authorized to provide the patient with a copy of their medical record?
   a. Registered nurse
   b. Medical provider
   c. Unit clerk
   d. Medical records administrator

33. The nurse manager observes a nurse struggling with time management. She appears busy throughout her shift and spends long periods of time working with her assigned patients. However, she has not been able to establish a system for when to document her patient care or take breaks. The nurse manager meets with the nurse and notes that she accrues overtime throughout the week. The nurse is advised to work within her scheduled hours. This is an example of:
   a. care delivery.
   b. conflict management.
   c. financial stewardship.
   d. staff engagement.

34. Which of the following describes type I diabetes?
   a. Manageable with dietary changes
   b. Complete or severe insufficiency of insulin production
   c. Typically appears during adulthood
   d. May not be lifelong

35. A new nurse is administering a blood thinner subcutaneously to a patient. The nurse injects the medication in the abdominal tissue, removes the syringe, and cannot determine how to activate the safety gauge. He fumbles with the syringe and mistakenly sticks himself with the needle. How should the nurse first proceed?
   a. Ask the patient if he is carrying an infectious pathogen.
   b. Wash the exposure with soap and water.
   c. File a safety report.
   d. Notify the charge nurse immediately.

36. C-Suite leadership is developing a strategy to combat implicit bias within the organization. What component should be included when developing training for their personnel?
   a. A one-time class on recognizing implicit bias
   b. Interactive training that includes a self-assessment for all staff and providers
   c. Comprehensive bias training that is delivered to the bedside staff
   d. Training that focuses on the micro levels of racial perceptions

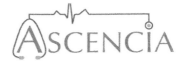

37. What is the primary focus of the Academy of Medical-Surgical Nurses (AMSN) Scope and Standards of Practice regarding the nursing role in providing interventions?
    a. Advocating for the patient's well-being while respecting their preferences and wishes
    b. Implementing interventions solely based on clinical evidence
    c. Prioritizing the nurse's recommendations over the patient's choices
    d. Fostering a one-sided approach to patient care

38. A speech therapist has administered a swallow test to a patient. The patient was able to swallow dry crackers and thickened liquids. What should occur next?
    a. The speech therapist should clear the patient for a regular diet
    b. The speech therapist should schedule a barium swallow study
    c. The speech therapist should ask the patient to speak after eating
    d. The speech therapist should order a consult for otolaryngology

39. The nurse manager receives consistent reports about an inaccurate narcotic count and suspects that one of his nurses is involved with drug diversion. He requests a meeting with the nurse in his office. When he discusses his findings with her, which of the following behaviors would be suspicious for drug diversion:
    a. A pain medication was retrieved 35 minutes prior to the medication administration time.
    b. Drugs that are required to be wasted are always immediately documented as wasted.
    c. When a patient reports pain, the nurse gives the smallest medication dose possible.
    d. According to the time clock, the nurse is always punctual and leaves on time.

40. When may additive or adjuvant treatment be added?
    a. Once the patient returns to baseline
    b. When it is determined that the current treatment is ineffective
    c. If the patient cannot tolerate the current treatment
    d. After an evaluation determines that the intervention was partially successful

41. The nurse is concerned with the nurse-patient ratio and feels that a reduced patient assignment could lead to better patient outcomes. She attends healthcare policy forums and speaks to her state legislature. The nurse knows that this is an example of:
    a. advocacy.
    b. autonomy.
    c. opposition.
    d. self-determination.

42. The nurse is caring for an 85-year-old male patient admitted with worsening confusion. He constantly attempts to get out of bed and yells out that he wants to go home. An unlicensed assistive personnel (UAP) is assigned to provide continuous monitoring of the patient. When the nurse makes rounds, she finds that the UAP has used a sheet across the patient's body to strap the patient to the bed. What is the nurse's immediate response?
    a. Remove the sheet from the bed.
    b. File a safety report so that the issue can be investigated.
    c. Contact the nurse manager to report the incident.
    d. Assess the patient's cognition.

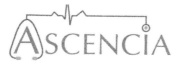

43. How can the interdisciplinary care team support patient autonomy and advocacy?
   a. By requesting social work to discuss post-hospitalization plans with the patient on the day of discharge
   b. By relaying information to the nurse to communicate with the patient and family
   c. By participating in bedside rounding with the patient and family as active members
   d. By encouraging nurses to deliver reports prior to meeting with the patient

44. A healthcare facility has activated the emergency response plan due to an internal chemical spill. The hospital incident command system (HCIS) is managing the disaster response. An incident commander is serving as the overall leader. The nurse understands that the role of allocating personnel resources in order to effectively respond to the disaster belongs to the:
   a. liaison officer.
   b. logistics officer.
   c. public information officer.
   d. security and safety officer.

45. The nurse has an assignment of four patients, each taking medications that produce notable side effects. When he begins his shift, which patient does he see FIRST?
   a. The 67-year-old male patient reporting humming in his ears after several doses of vancomycin
   b. The 56-year-old female patient with a temperature of 101.1°F after receiving her first dose of amoxicillin
   c. The 86-year-old female patient with a blood pressure of 180/90, 30 minutes after taking losartan
   d. The 48-year-old male patient reporting diarrhea after taking lactulose

46. The nurse is preparing a patient who has a tracheostomy tube with a cuff to eat. Which of the following will assist in preventing aspiration?
   a. Inflating the cuff fully
   b. Drinking frequent sips of thin liquids
   c. Taking larger bites
   d. Chewing food 20 times prior to attempting to swallow

47. Which of the following consequences of an unhealthy workplace environment is characterized by emotional exhaustion, depersonalization, and reduced personal accomplishment, often resulting from chronic workplace stress?
   a. Moral distress and moral injuries
   b. Compassion fatigue
   c. Burnout
   d. Job dissatisfaction

48. A facility is distributing smart IV pumps to the med-surg unit. How does this technology best support safe medication administration?
   a. Controlled delivery of intravenous solutions
   b. Updated drug formulary with set limits
   c. Lock-out options to deter patients from changing rates
   d. Adjustable volume to prevent alarm fatigue

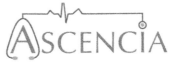

49. The nurse is caring for an 82-year-old male patient admitted for altered mental status and agitation. He is oriented to person only but at baseline is oriented to person and place. After he is treated for a urinary tract infection, his cognition returns to his baseline, and he is ready for discharge. His daughter is concerned about the patient's progressively worsening memory loss and would like information on how to store his medication at home. The nurse includes all of the following about medication storage, EXCEPT:
   a. Most medications should be stored in a specific temperature range of 59–86°F (15–30°C).
   b. The patient's pills should be kept out of reach in a locked medicine cabinet in the bathroom.
   c. Oral tablets should be kept in their original container with the label instructions.
   d. The environment is very important because sunlight often affects medication effectiveness.

50. The nurse is taking care of a Hispanic patient on a regular diet who has been eating poorly. He states that he is just not that hungry and is missing home meals. What intervention by the nurse may encourage the patient to eat?
   a. Request that family bring in some foods from home
   b. Bring the patient some protein shakes to try
   c. Notify the provider that the patient is non-compliant with their diet
   d. Suggest that the patient order something in from a restaurant if he does not like hospital food

51. The organization is undergoing a system-wide disaster recovery plan and providing education to the nursing staff. One of the topics is cybersecurity. The education includes unplanned downtime procedures if there is a computer system threat. The nurse understands that an active role to prevent a cybersecurity risk and protect patient safety includes which of the following actions?
   a. Clarifying an order by texting complete information to an ordering physician including name and date of birth
   b. Always logging out of charting systems prior to leaving the work station
   c. Rescheduling a prompted computer update, as this is the responsibility of an Information Technology (IT) staff member
   d. Using a password that is used for other logins to prevent forgetting login information

52. A newly licensed nurse enters nursing as a second career after caring for her brother who was dying of cancer. She was inspired by one of his nurses who provided care for her brother with dignity and encouraged him to make decisions, even when he was not able to do the activities that he once could. The newly licensed nurse is excited and passionate about helping patients to feel that level of respect. She explains these sentiments in her cover letter for a nursing position. This testimony is best described as:
   a. clinical judgment.
   b. nursing ethics.
   c. nursing philosophy.
   d. compassionate care.

53. Communication among the interdisciplinary team helps to:
   a. provide comprehensive care.
   b. drive disease-focused care.
   c. decrease the amount of potentially troubling information that is relayed to the patient.
   d. create a silo of information within a specialty department.

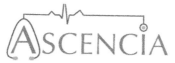

54. When is the most advantageous time for the patient to be approached regarding advance directives?
  a. With any clinical or office encounter or admission to a hospital
  b. When scheduled for surgery
  c. During a clinical emergency
  d. When the patient is diagnosed with a terminal illness

55. What is the primary goal of emotional workplace safety in nursing, and why is it essential for healthcare professionals?
  a. The primary goal of emotional workplace safety is to eliminate all workplace challenges for healthcare professionals, ensuring a stress-free environment.
  b. The primary goal of emotional workplace safety is to maintain physical well-being and minimize the need for adaptation in healthcare settings.
  c. The primary goal of emotional workplace safety is to provide a workplace culture where healthcare professionals can express their opinions without any limitations.
  d. The primary goal of emotional workplace safety is to ensure the psychological and emotional well-being of healthcare professionals by creating a supportive workplace culture.

56. Which of the following is forbidden in a kosher diet?
  a. Beef
  b. Lobster
  c. Dairy
  d. Chicken

57. A 45-year-old male patient is admitted to the medical unit after sustaining a fall with injury. He reports significant pain and requires pain medication. The nurse knows that the ordered medication is given via IV push, one of the routes that puts the patient at the greatest risk of harm because of its immediate bioavailability. The best way that she can avoid patient harm is:
  a. reconstituting the medication using aseptic technique in the medication room.
  b. looking in her institutional drug reference guide for the rate of administration.
  c. transferring the proper medication dose from the vial into a sterile syringe.
  d. diluting the medication with 0.9% normal saline.

58. The nurse is preparing to administer parenteral nutrition to a patient. Which of the following vascular access lines is the gold standard for administering this alternative nutrition?
  a. Mid-line
  b. PICC
  c. IV
  d. PEG

59. The nurse is admitting a 19-year-old female to the nursing unit who has injuries related to a motor vehicle incident. She has a laceration to her forehead, a bloody stain on her shirt, and torn pants. The patient appears anxious and fearful. She does not speak much English and is accompanied by an older man who is able to answer the nurse's questions. Which action is LEAST warranted by the nurse?
  a. Schedule an appointment with an approved translator.
  b. Perform a comprehensive assessment.
  c. Ask the man to stay in the room to allay the patient's anxiety.
  d. Use open-ended questions to elicit responses.

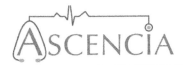

60. What is the risk of not fully capturing clinical care documentation?
   a. Improved accessibility to health information
   b. Poor patient outcomes
   c. Improved treatment decisions
   d. Increased time management

61. The nurse is preparing her 75-year-old female patient's morning medication pass. When he removes all of the medications from the automated dispensing cabinet, he counts that the patient is receiving 14 medications in total. He is concerned about the quantity of drugs because he knows that polypharmacy can lead to drug-drug interactions. The nurse knows that all of the following statements about polypharmacy are true EXCEPT:
   a. Prescribers may need to order additional medication to manage side effects.
   b. A greater effect of a particular drug may be experienced when more than one medication is administered.
   c. There is less of a potential for side effects when the patient can take their medications all at once.
   d. The nurse may need to assess the patient's fall risk and implement fall precautions.

62. Which of the following statements best describes a dependent nursing intervention?
   a. It is team oriented.
   b. It is within the nurse's scope of practice.
   c. It involves multiple disciplines to coordinate.
   d. It is ordered by an advanced practice provider.

63. The nurse manager observes the change-of-shift throughout the week. A few months ago, the organization engaged in a large initiative for nurses to provide handoffs at the bedside to improve patient satisfaction and safety. He discovered that most staff are providing bedside handoffs, although he is frustrated because several nurses are still giving shift reports at the nurse's station. Using the ADKAR change model, what step does the nurse manager need to take next?
   a. Call a staff meeting and recognize the nurses he observed providing bedside handoffs.
   b. Determine which shift bedside handoff could be trialed to identify any adjustments that are needed.
   c. Create awareness among the staff that there is a need to change shift reports to bedside handoff.
   d. Ask the nurse educator to set up in-services for the staff on the importance of bedside handoff.

64. A feeding pump is alarming during the delivery of enteral formula via a nasogastric tube. Why is it important for the nurse to immediately stop the pump and assess the patient?
   a. The patient may be overfed.
   b. The formula might be leaking from the tubing.
   c. There is a high risk of aspiration to the patient.
   d. A flow stoppage may affect the electronics of the device.

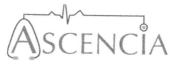

65. The nurse is caring for a Jewish patient who has requested a meal of roast beef, mashed potatoes, and a cup of milk. The nurse is concerned that the order is mistaken. What is the best action for the nurse to take?
   a.   Change the order for the drink to a non-dairy product
   b.   Ensure that the milk is not served on the same tray
   c.   Ask the patient if there are any preferences regarding their order
   d.   Leave the order as it is

66. The nurse is caring for a patient diagnosed with Crohn's disease who had a peripherally inserted central catheter (PICC) line inserted one week ago. He reports feeling tired, with discomfort at the PICC site, and the nurse suspects a central line-associated bloodstream infection (CLABSI). What sign would best indicate to the nurse that the patient has a complication?
   a.   Fatigue
   b.   Respiratory rate of 20 breaths/minute
   c.   Temperature of 100.5 °F
   d.   Urinary output of 20 mL/hr

67. The nurse is delegating the task of oral care to a nursing assistant. Which statement is most true about delegation?
   a.   The nurse is ultimately accountable for the task being completed.
   b.   The nursing assistant is responsible for determining the patient's needs.
   c.   The nurse determines the nursing responsibilities that can be delegated.
   d.   The nursing assistant must accept the task if she is busy.

68. Why is it important to clarify roles within an interdisciplinary team?
   a.   To decrease the amount of reporting
   b.   To ensure that all members of the team round together
   c.   To respond to emergencies more effectively
   d.   To ensure that roles are kept separate and establish hierarchy

69. The nurse is caring for a 55-year-old patient and was surprised to receive a newly prescribed order for warfarin 5 mg daily. What is the nurse's priority action before administering the medication?
   a.   Ask the patient for his name and date of birth prior to using the barcode scanner.
   b.   Request a dietician consult so that the patient receives information about foods to avoid with vitamin K.
   c.   Contact the pharmacy to verify that the patient is receiving the proper dose for initiating therapy.
   d.   Speak with the ordering provider about the indication for use.

70. A patient who had jaw restructuring surgery has progressed to being able to intake food by mouth. The nurse has administered an initial swallow study; the patient was able to swallow applesauce but choked on crackers. What is the next best step?
   a.   Repeat the swallow study the following day.
   b.   Allow the patient to eat applesauce.
   c.   Notify the provider that the patient needs the NG tube converted to a gastronomy tube.
   d.   Request an order for a barium swallow study.

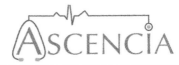

71. What is the first step the nurse informaticist will take when addressing a problem in the documentation process?
    a. Apply a modification
    b. Review results
    c. Analyze the issue
    d. Implement an intervention

72. The nurse has placed a nasogastric tube in a patient who has an order for enteral nutrition. Which of the following is the best practice for verifying appropriate placement?
    a. pH > 6
    b. Chest x-ray
    c. Air bolus auscultation above epigastric space
    d. Because the procedure was well tolerated and the tube placed easily, no verification is required

73. To respond most effectively to a disaster, the hospital is evaluating hazards to ensure that the organization's operations will run smoothly during a crisis. The nurse understands that this phase is called:
    a. mitigation.
    b. modification.
    c. planning.
    d. preparedness.

74. The nurse sees a new order for a heparin IV infusion. When she enters the medication room to retrieve the medication, she notices a sticker indicating that the medication is "high-alert." She knows that this is especially important because:
    a. baseline labs, including a PTT, will need to be ordered for monitoring if the patient's blood is too thin.
    b. an independent double check is required prior to medication administration.
    c. heparin is a medication with a high potential for error.
    d. heparin is a medication that requires dosage calculations according to the patient's weight.

75. What occurs if a care plan does not meet all outcomes?
    a. The current treatment continues until all outcomes are met.
    b. The care plan is revisited and adjusted.
    c. The patient's disease process is deemed incurable.
    d. The care plan is discontinued.

76. A nurse observes a colleague from another healthcare discipline completing a procedure that is clearly outside their authorized scope of practice. What should the nurse do in this situation?
    a. The nurse should confront the colleague immediately and instruct them to stop the procedure.
    b. The nurse should report the incident to their immediate supervisor or charge nurse.
    c. The nurse should ignore the situation, as it does not directly involve their own practice.
    d. The nurse should provide assistance to the colleague to ensure the procedure is completed safely.

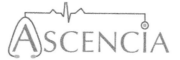

77. Which of the following documentation modifications would support a safer patient experience?
    a. Increasing the number of computer clicks
    b. Reducing the availability of shortcuts
    c. Allowing providers to easily override hard stops
    d. Providing visual clues to prompt action

78. The nurse manager is concerned about the nurse turnover on her unit due to increasing conflict and poor morale. She is looking for strategies for improving job engagement and retention. What is a method she could use?
    a. Increase interest in certification by including it as a mandatory part of performance evaluation.
    b. Ask a newer nurse to represent the unit by participating in a work environment committee.
    c. Address the conflict right away and reprimand the staff who do not comply with the policies.
    d. Require staff to attend education on ways to deal with managing conflicts.

79. How can healthcare providers most effectively address a patient's expectations?
    a. By promising patients that their care team will provide the highest quality care in the nation
    b. By telling the nursing staff to treat certain patients as VIP status
    c. By establishing reasonable goals upon admission
    d. By providing service recovery as soon as a concern is voiced by the patient

80. The nurse has established a nursing diagnosis of acute pain related to myocardial infarction, as evidenced by chest pain, pallor, ECG changes, and diaphoresis. What would be the priority intervention for this diagnosis?
    a. Administering supplemental oxygen
    b. Preparing the patient for percutaneous coronary intervention
    c. Delivering intravenous fibrinolytic therapy
    d. Checking blood sugar levels

81. The nurse is assisting a nursing coworker with the care of a new surgical patient. The patient wishes to get out of bed and has orders to do so. The coworker decides to administer the patient's scheduled subcutaneous heparin prior to mobilizing him. Upon completing the medication administration, the nurse observes her coworker using her fingers to push the safety device over the needle. How should the nurse first respond?
    a. "I am concerned that you will stick yourself. I am going to report you to the nurse manager for not complying with sharps safety procedures."
    b. "I am concerned that you will stick yourself. I would like to show you how to correctly engage the safety device."
    c. "I am concerned that you will stick yourself. I will ask the nurse educator to review how to engage the sharps safety device."
    d. The nurse does not need to say anything to her coworker.

82. The nurse is taking care of a patient who has started slurring speech spontaneously. She assesses the patient for signs of a cerebral vascular accident. Which of the following is considered a classic sign of a stroke?
    a. Facial asymmetry
    b. Spastic movements
    c. Throat pain
    d. Chest pain

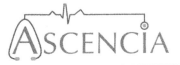

83. What is the first step in the nursing process?
   a.   Diagnosis
   b.   Assessment
   c.   Implementation
   d.   Planning

84. What is the most effective way to ensure that an oropharyngeal tube is correctly placed?
   a.   pH test
   b.   Auscultation of air bolus
   c.   Aspiration of gastric fluid
   d.   Chest x-ray

85. The nurse manager of a medical-surgical nursing unit is looking for ways to reduce staff turnover and improve retention. She is going to implement a mentorship program for newly hired nurses and surveyed experienced staff about a desire to mentor. During the education provided, the nurse manager explained that the mentor-mentee relationship is best described as:
   a.   a specified amount of time that allows the mentor to assess the mentee's competence.
   b.   a long-term professional relationship that enhances growth and development.
   c.   a short-term arrangement that encourages self-assessment and reflection.
   d.   a long-term relationship that sets aside time for the mentee to teach.

86. The nurse is providing discharge instructions to a patient returning home following a total knee replacement. The nurse asks the patient to describe the home environment to determine any safety needs. Which findings would warrant further follow-up?
   a.   The patient reports one step into the house.
   b.   The home contains hardwood floors throughout.
   c.   The patient grabs a towel rack to help sit on the toilet.
   d.   The patient has primarily frozen food stocked up.

87. The nurse attends an interprofessional committee representing her nursing unit. The discussion topic is ways to mitigate medication error and patient harm. The members want to ensure that there are safeguards to reduce risk. The following strategies are discussed, EXCEPT:
   a.   Standardizing the preparation of total parenteral nutrition
   b.   Ensuring that nurses have easy access to high-alert medications
   c.   Purchasing a drug reference guide that would be available from the electronic medication administration record
   d.   Affixing a brightly colored alert label on the IV heparin solution

88. A patient newly diagnosed with celiac disease is receiving dietary education on meal planning. Which of the following meal choices would indicate that the patient understands their dietary limitation?
   a.   Roast beef and cheddar sandwich on a brioche roll with an apple
   b.   Chicken taco with corn tortillas and salsa
   c.   Beef and barley soup with a side salad and ranch dressing
   d.   Blueberry oatmeal muffin with a glass of milk

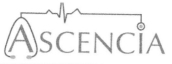

89. What is one of the responsibilities that patients typically have as part of their healthcare experience?
    a. The right to informed consent
    b. The right to voice grievances
    c. Providing accurate medical information
    d. Access to medical records

90. The nurse is caring for a patient diagnosed with influenza. The patient reports a sore throat, fatigue, and body aches. He is actively coughing with copious amounts of sputum production. Upon entering the patient's room, the nurse discovers the patient's daughter sitting at his bedside. What is the best response of the nurse?
    a. "Your father is very infectious. You will need to leave immediately."
    b. "You will need to wear a gown and gloves when you sit at the bedside. Place the gown on by securely fastening it and making sure the fabric fully covers your arms and torso. Then, put the gloves on with the openings covering the edge of the gown."
    c. "You should be careful of your father's cough. The droplets can suspend in the air and fall within two feet."
    d. "You will need to wear a gown, goggles, a mask, and gloves around your father. The gown must be fastened and cover your torso. Next, the mask is placed, ensuring a snug fit across your nose to your chin. Place the goggles over your eyes and then put on the gloves, with the openings covering the edge of the gown."

91. The nurse is caring for an oriented 83-year-old female patient admitted for a pleural effusion. The patient reports difficulty breathing, and the nurse administers newly ordered furosemide. Later in the shift, the nurse walks into the patient room and finds the patient on the floor. The initial nursing assessment does not show any injury. A few hours later, the patient's speech is slurred, and she is confused. A CT scan reveals a subdural hematoma. The nurse best describes this situation as:
    a. an adverse event because the patient fell as a result of feeling dizzy after receiving furosemide.
    b. a side effect from furosemide because the patient experienced urinary urgency and tried to get up by herself.
    c. a root cause because the furosemide was administered as a result of the pleural effusion.
    d. a sentinel event because the patient experienced injury unrelated to the pleural effusion.

92. The nurse has planned an intervention based on a nursing diagnosis. Which of the following is true regarding a nursing diagnosis?
    a. It is the same as a medical diagnosis.
    b. It focuses on the disease and aims to treat the signs and symptoms.
    c. It is a standard and peer-reviewed recommendation.
    d. Is used to guide the primary treatment of the patient.

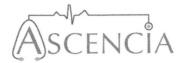

93. A nurse manager is in a situation where he has to manage the conflict between a nurse and a nursing assistant. The nursing assistant needs help with mobilizing a patient, but the nurse does not want to help because she often finds the nursing assistant in the corner of the hallway not responding to call lights. After meeting with the nurse manager, the nurse agrees to help get the patient out of bed and the nursing assistant agrees to answer call lights. This conflict management style that facilitates a quick solution requiring two staff members to meet in the middle is called:
   a. accommodating.
   b. collaborating.
   c. competing.
   d. compromising.

94. What is a central tenet of nursing ethics emphasized in the Nursing Code of Ethics?
   a. Ensuring the financial well-being of healthcare institutions
   b. Safeguarding patient autonomy and advocating for their best interests
   c. Expediting healthcare procedures to minimize costs
   d. Prioritizing healthcare providers' convenience and comfort

95. The nurse is caring for a 36-year-old male admitted for acute pancreatitis. He has a long history of alcohol use and chronic pain. The healthcare provider has ordered morphine IV for pain every 4 hours PRN for pain management. The nurse feels frustrated because the patient uses his call light and requests pain medication 30 minutes before the medication is due. The nurse delays answering the call light because she suspects he is abusing narcotics. How does this situation best describe the nurse?
   a. Moral disengagement
   b. Principle of nonmaleficence
   c. Intentional tort
   d. Paternalism

96. A provider is preparing to meet with a patient for the first time. What technique would help the patient feel more comfortable during the clinical visit?
   a. Having an interpreter available since the patient is listed as Hispanic in the chart
   b. Standing while the patient is sitting to show confidence
   c. Interrupting while the patient is talking to seek clarification in the moment
   d. Facing the patient and maintaining comfortable eye contact

97. An IV pump is not functioning as expected. What is the best action by the nurse?
   a. Use it until another one can be obtained
   b. Place it in the supply closet
   c. Remove from service and submit a repair ticket
   d. Throw it in the biohazardous waste container

98. The nurse is admitting a patient to the medical-surgical unit and is verifying their history. Which of the following is the primary source for this information?
   a. Family members
   b. Previous caregivers
   c. Family care provider
   d. Patient

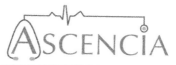

99. A 36-year-old female patient is admitted for a wound abscess that requires antibiotics. The patient reports to the nurse that she is not able to afford her medications. The nurse knows that she will need to bring this concern to the interdisciplinary team because:

    a.   the healthcare provider will be able to prescribe brand-name drugs that are cheaper for the patient.

    b.   the insurance company needs to be alerted that the patient cannot afford any copay.

    c.   the patient may not take all of the medication as the physician prescribed.

    d.   the antibiotic will need to be discontinued before the patient is discharged.

100. The nurse is evaluating the effectiveness of the interventions put in place for a patient with shortness of breath and decreased oxygen levels. A goal set in the planning stage was that the patient would maintain an oxygen saturation of > 92% on 3 L of supplemental O_2. What element of a SMART goal is missing?

    a.   Time-based

    b.   Measurable

    c.   Specific

    d.   Achievable

101. A patient is admitted to the medical-surgical unit after undergoing a right hip ORIF as a result of a fall. The patient was ambulatory prior to admission. On postoperative day 3, the nurse plans to assist the patient out of bed and the patient replies, "I have not been out of bed yet." The nurse reviews the electronic record and notes the physician order for ambulation after surgery, but does not see any nursing documentation about the patient's mobility. The nurse enters a safety report, and the nurse manager decides to refer the issue to a professional nurse committee that enhances self-regulation. This committee is called:

    a.   nursing peer evaluation.

    b.   nursing peer review.

    c.   nursing administrative evaluation.

    d.   nursing policy review.

102. What evidence-based key initiative dictated the implementation, minimum standards, and widespread use of electronic medical records?

    a.   HIPAA

    b.   Healthy People 2030

    c.   Meaningful Use

    d.   Equitable Long-Term Recovery and Resilience

103. A nurse is very engaged in professional development. He constantly seeks new knowledge by attending education and seminars, and he volunteers for committees and values feedback. He explains to his colleague that a group of abilities involving growth in his knowledge, skills, and thinking when performing his nursing duties is called:

    a.   aptitude.

    b.   capability.

    c.   competence.

    d.   competencies.

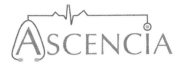

104. Which of the following is an effect of interdisciplinary collaboration and communication?
    a.   Decreased interruptions
    b.   Intermittent critical thinking
    c.   Improved patient outcomes
    d.   Increased patient acuity

105. A preceptor is teaching a newly licensed nurse about how to administer a piggy-back antibiotic through an IV pump. The preceptor explains the procedure to the preceptee with detailed instructions, but the new nurse feels overwhelmed. Next, she shows the preceptee how to insert the tubing into the IV pump using clean supplies. When the nurse still does not understand, the preceptor draws a picture. The preceptee exclaimed, "Now I get it!" Of the following selections, which learning style does she most prefer?
    a.   Auditory
    b.   Kinesthetic
    c.   Reading
    d.   Visual

106. A med-surg nurse is preparing to teach a patient with several socioeconomic disparities about the intake of sufficient dietary nutrients. Which of the following may be a barrier?
    a.   Access to a local grocery store
    b.   High reliance on convenience food
    c.   No noted disabilities
    d.   Urban dwelling

107. A healthcare system reorganized its leadership. A nurse manager met with her nursing staff and described that the purpose of her role was best described as:
    a.   overseeing multiple medical-surgical nursing units.
    b.   directing and coordinating the workflow during the shift.
    c.   running the daily operations of the nursing unit.
    d.   establishing the nursing strategic plan.

108. The nurse is caring for a seventy-five-year-old male admitted for a diabetic wound infection on his right foot. He is ordered to receive IV piperacillin-tazobactam and states that he has experienced severe diarrhea from an antimicrobial in the past. He asks the nurse what type of food could help prevent this. Which of the following selections does the nurse include in his teaching?
    a.   Kefir, yogurt, kombucha
    b.   Chicken, beans, whole wheat bread
    c.   Apples, eggs, whole milk
    d.   Cooked potatoes, white rice, bananas

109. What lab value should be closely monitored during the first 72 hours of TPN administration?
    a.   Blood glucose
    b.   Sodium
    c.   Potassium
    d.   WBC

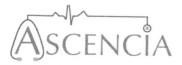

110. An unexpected tornado affected the area of a regional hospital. The emergency response plan is activated and physical space is arranged to accommodate a large number of patients. Patients are being transferred for emergent care. Which patient does the nurse prioritize when triaging?
   a. A patient who was hit in the torso with a large branch and sustained several superficial lacerations to the chest
   b. A patient who reports feeling panicky with chest pain, tachypnea, and palpitations
   c. A patient who was trying to run from the chaos, slipped on wet ground, and reports that his foot twisted in an odd position
   d. A patient who was knocked over by a flying object, sustained an open fracture of his arm, and has a distal pulse

111. A newly licensed nurse is orienting with a preceptor on a medical-surgical nursing unit. As part of his orientation, an observation day in the operating room (OR) is planned. After entering the OR, the nurse is introduced to all of the members of the surgical team. One nursing member is responsible for conducting a preoperative nursing assessment, handling certain surgical instruments, and providing hemostasis. The nurse learns that this member is called the:
   a. registered nurse circulator.
   b. registered nurse first assistant.
   c. surgical scrub nurse.
   d. vascular access nurse.

112. When a charge nurse starts her shift, she discovers that two nursing assistants called out sick and there is no replacement help. Many of the patients require full assistance with bathing and feeding. She requests a huddle and explains the situation to the staff. She asks for input on how the unit can effectively manage the workload for the shift. What type of leadership style is the charge nurse using?
   a. Autocratic
   b. Democratic
   c. Laissez-faire
   d. Transformational

113. The nurse responds to an IV pump alarm. What should the nurse first do?
   a. Assess for kinks in the IV tubing
   b. Ask the patient if they were touching the buttons
   c. Pause the IV pump
   d. Ensure the pump is plugged in

114. What is a major cause of heart failure exacerbation?
   a. Excess sodium intake
   b. Occasional alcohol consumption
   c. Diuretic usage
   d. Fluid-restricted diet

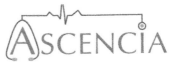

115. The nurse is caring for a 65-year-old female admitted for chest pain, and the tests rule out a myocardial infarction. The patient has her call light on and reports to the nurse that she has mild chest pain. The nurse obtains nitroglycerin and performs the five rights of medication administration. After she opens the package, she notes that the doctor discontinued the nitroglycerin and ordered aluminum hydroxide instead. In which location does the nurse decide to waste the nitroglycerin?

    a. Down the toilet before leaving the patient room.
    b. In the nonhazardous pharmaceutical waste bin.
    c. In the hazardous pharmaceutical waste bin.
    d. In the bin that denatures the pharmaceutical drug.

116. Which of the following would be considered objective data?

    a. Pain described as throbbing
    b. Feeling dizzy
    c. Blood loss of 30 mL
    d. Nausea

117. A newly licensed nurse has a patient assignment for the first time. Halfway through the shift, the patient codes and is unable to be resuscitated. The nurse manager decides to meet with the nurse to debrief right after the event. She provides a calm environment, asks for details about what happened, actively listens, and encourages the nurse to share their emotions. What leadership role is the nurse manager providing?

    a. Advocacy
    b. Autonomy
    c. Compliance
    d. Resource utilization

118. Which of the following vitamin deficiencies is most commonly caused by lack of dairy intake?

    a. Calciferol
    b. Magnesium
    c. Riboflavin
    d. Ascorbic acid

119. What is the purpose of an organization participating in watchdog data collection?

    a. To perform auditing and observation to identify deficiencies in patient care areas
    b. To gather patient feedback via surveys
    c. To collect information on underperforming staff
    d. To provide quality reviews after a sentinel event

120. A preceptor is teaching a preceptee about clinical judgment. She explains to the newly licensed nurse that clinical judgment has to do with interpreting the patient's needs and deciding the next action step. Which statement would NOT describe clinical judgment?

    a. Clinical judgment is a systematic process involving assessment, planning, implementation, and evaluation.
    b. Clinical judgment uses observation of patterns and a strong knowledge-base.
    c. Clinical judgment takes into consideration previous encounters with prior patients.
    d. Clinical judgment involves the ability to reflect upon the patient interactions within the nurse-patient relationship.

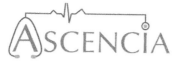

121. What information is appropriate to include on an inpatient whiteboard?
   a. Mobility status
   b. Noncompliance issues
   c. Insurance information
   d. Social Security number

122. A newly licensed nurse is hired to work on a medical-surgical nursing unit. In order to complete his training, the nurse is assigned to a preceptor during his orientation. He is told that the preceptor is a nurse who also works on the unit and has a few years of experience. The nurse understands that the role of the preceptor is best described as:
   a. deepening the preceptee's professional development.
   b. encouraging the preceptee with his communication skills.
   c. assessing the preceptee's ability to perform care.
   d. introducing the preceptee to the nursing unit staff.

123. The renal system has many important functions. Which of the following is NOT a function provided by the kidneys?
   a. Maintaining pH balance through H+ buffer system
   b. Regulating blood pressure
   c. Filtering byproduct waste
   d. Assisting with protein breakdown

124. A nurse is seeking a way to contribute to elevating patient safety and nursing education at a national level. Which of the following is the best method to achieve these goals?
   a. Reading nursing journals on patient safety topics
   b. Enrolling in a BSN program to achieve a higher degree
   c. Being a keynote speaker at a televised conference on preventing patient harm
   d. Running for a political position with goals of improving healthcare policy aimed at patient safety

125. How does palliative care differ from hospice care?
   a. Hospice care is aimed at curative care along with promoting comfort
   b. Palliative care is for end-of-life when no further measures are desired
   c. Hospice care aims to alleviate pain and discomfort when all treatments have been exhausted
   d. A patient can choose hospice care regardless of diagnosis, but palliative care must be ordered by a healthcare provider

Answer Explanations #1

1. C: The correct answer is Choice *C*. A CAUTI bundle is implemented as an infection prevention tool, providing standardized care practices for patients with an indwelling urinary catheter in place. The nurse should assess the necessity of the catheter daily to ensure that it is removed as soon as medically appropriate. The catheter should be maintained BELOW the level of the bladder, not on an IV pole. The insertion site is cleansed with hospital-approved soap and water, not hospital-grade disinfecting wipes. Lastly, urine collection bags should not be changed on a scheduled basis. This breaks the closed system. Urine collection bags should be changed as medically indicated.

2. B: The correct answer is Choice *B*. The newly admitted patient diagnosed with dysphagia following a stroke is at high risk for aspiration, which could lead to a number of complications such as pneumonia, acute respiratory distress syndrome, and mortality. If the patient is not able to swallow, then he should be maintained NPO until a speech evaluation is complete.

3. A: The correct answer is Choice *A*; dieticians must monitor a patient's metabolic needs closely with acute clinical processes—such as injury or fever—because caloric needs increase greatly as metabolic catabolism increases demand for energy. Choice *B* is incorrect because the system is not able to meet demand on its own, especially with a critical illness occurring. Choice *C* is not correct because metabolic demand increases, not decreases, caloric needs. Choice *D* is incorrect because a lowered insulin production does not allow glucose to be transported into the cells, leading to hyperglycemia.

4. C: In the context of maintaining adequate physical resources for workplace safety in nursing practice, ensuring proper hand hygiene protocols is not directly associated with physical resources, but rather with personal hygiene practices. Although hand hygiene is crucial for infection control and patient safety, it is not considered a physical resource like the other options. Choice *A* involves proper equipment and procedures to ensure the safe disposal of hazardous materials. Choice *B* ensures that equipment is in proper working condition, which is essential for maintaining a safe healthcare environment. Choice *D* pertains to staffing levels and resource allocation, which are critical for patient safety and quality care.

5. D: The correct answer is Choice *D*. Once the nurse steps away from the bedside, she must identify the patient again by asking him for his name and date of birth and verifying that he is the right person with the medication administration record.

6. A: Choice *A* is correct, as subjective and objective data is used to determine the efficacy of an intervention to meet goals and outcomes. Choice *B* does not evaluate whether there was a clinical change in the patient's condition; the patient may feel better solely from improved pain control rather than treatment of the disease process. Choice *C* is incorrect, as it is not patient centered and does not include evaluative data from the patient's perspective. In Choice *D*, some outcomes are met, not all; therefore, the outcomes should be revisited to determine whether further intervention is needed to meet the deficits in goals.

7. A: The correct answer is Choice *A* as this improves patient care by minimizing medical errors through decreasing duplicate orders that could lead to a patient receiving inappropriate, duplicate care. Choice *B* is incorrect as communication should be encouraged and enhanced to improve patient-centered care.

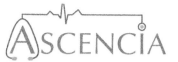

Choice *C* is incorrect because information should be delivered in a timely manner to guide in-the-moment care. Choice *D* is incorrect as duplicate claims are fraudulent.

8. A: The correct answer is Choice *A*. The goal of the early phase of recovery is recovery from anesthesia and restoration of baseline vital signs. Preparing for the patient discharge to home occurs in the late phase (PACU phase 2). Patients who are intubated will often be transferred to the critical care unit. Dysphagia screening occurs to identify aspiration postoperatively but does not describe the early phase.

9. C: The correct answer is Choice *C*. The nurse should suspect *Clostridium difficile* and plan the patient's care accordingly. Contact precautions should be implemented to reduce the potential of organism transmission. While the doctor should be notified and a stool specimen sent to the lab for confirmation, the initial priority is to prevent exposure to a suspected transmittable disease. The diarrhea is a side effect of the medication and not the result of an allergy.

10. C: The correct answer is Choice *C*; it is recommended that individuals with kidney failure should limit sodium intake to less than 2000 milligrams per day. This can prevent hypertensive effects that in turn cause further kidney damage.

11. D: The correct answer is Choice *D*. Once the nurse has delegated the task, she must monitor the completion of the assignment in order to evaluate the patient outcome. Confirming the documentation of the results refers to the right supervision.

12. B: Choice *B* is correct, as the patient's symptoms require a brief, systems-specific assessment that quickly evaluates the cardiac system to rule out a cardiovascular emergency. Choices *A* and *D* are thorough assessments that look at each body system; they are incorrect because this is more information than is needed to address the immediate concern. Choice *C* is not correct because the patient's symptoms are related to cardiovascular health, not cognitive function.

13. C: The correct answer is Choice *C*; the patient's reliance on purging with laxatives can cause electrolyte imbalances—especially with potassium, which may lead to life-threatening rhythms. Choices *A*, *B*, and *D* are not immediate threats to the patient's health status and are due to long-term malnutrition.

14. A: The correct answer is Choice *A*. The action that best supports antimicrobial stewardship is to talk with the medical provider and determine if the patient could be transitioned to an oral route of administration. The nurse would not need to obtain a sputum culture once the antibiotic has been administered. Although asking the patient to confirm his allergies would be appropriate with general nursing care, allergies for his treatment should have been determined prior to initiating the medication.

15. B: Choice *B* is correct, as the patient must be reevaluated to assess current symptoms and determine any efficacy of the failed intervention and whether there is any clinical change. This assessment should provide data to guide further diagnosis and intervention. Choices *A*, *C*, and *D* will be determined by the reassessment.

16. C: The correct answer is Choice *C*. The Board of Nursing for each state outlines the scope of practice for the LPN.

17. A: The correct answer is Choice *A*, as facility policy or order will determine the telemetry lead placement most appropriate based on the client's cardiovascular diagnosis. Choice *B* is a contraindication to the use of ECG electrodes as it prevents adherence. Choice *C* is incorrect as the hair should be clipped first to ensure full contact with the skin. Unless Choice *D*, the intermittent removal of telemetry leads, is specified in the order, the patient should not be taken off the monitoring device.

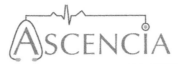

18. D: The answer is Choice *D*. In order to admit many new patients due to a disaster, patients who are stable would be discharged in order to make space available. Participating in mock drills and assessing community risks would be done prior to the disaster. Supporting the victims' psychological and emotional needs occurs after the disaster.

19. D: The Joint Commission is a key organization responsible for accrediting healthcare facilities and overseeing their adherence to safety and quality standards. This accreditation is a significant indicator of a facility's commitment to maintaining high standards of patient care and safety. Choice *A* is incorrect because the American Nurses Association (ANA) is responsible for developing the Nursing Code of Ethics and providing professional guidelines but is not involved in accrediting healthcare facilities. Choice *B* is incorrect because the State Board of Nursing is responsible for enforcing the Nurse Practice Act and regulating nursing licenses within a specific state but does not accredit healthcare facilities. Choice *C* is incorrect because the Centers for Medicare & Medicaid Services (CMS) administers critical federal healthcare programs and sets regulations that impact reimbursement, quality measurement, and patient safety in facilities that accept Medicare and Medicaid funding.

20. D: The correct answer is Choice *D* because the patient's immediate physical needs take precedence to ensure patient safety and comfort. While all these answers are correct, the nurse needs to FIRST address the patient and provide adequate care. Next, the case would be reported according to state laws/facility protocol and the social worker would be notified. If the son is involved with neglect, the priority of the nurse is to make certain that the patient is in a safe environment.

21. D: The correct answer is Choice *D*. Newly admitted patients are considered unstable. The nurse must first assess the patient's clinical condition. In this instance, the delegation of vital signs to the nursing assistant would not be appropriate.

22. D: The correct answer is Choice *D*. The surgical team jointly agrees upon the patient identification, surgical site, and procedure. The other options are not correct. The pre-procedure verification is mostly completed while the patient is awake. The timeout is conducted with the surgical team that will be present at the start of surgery. The pre-surgical checklist is initiated by the medical-surgical nurse.

23. C: The correct answer is Choice *C* as the real-time that the assessment occurred provides the most accurate timing to be referenced within the medical record. Choices *A*, *B*, and *D* do not reflect the time that the assessment occurred. Entries in the chart should be as close to real-time as possible or back-timed to reflect the time the assessment was completed.

24. A: One of the key steps in service recovery that reinforces the commitment to patient-centered care is the recognition of the issue and immediate corrective actions. This step demonstrates responsiveness to patient concerns and a proactive approach to resolving issues promptly. Choice *B* also represents a valid step in service recovery, but it does not specifically address the commitment to patient-centered care. Choices *C* and *D* are incorrect because they do not align with the principles of effective service recovery and patient-centered care.

25. B: The correct answer is Choice *B* as tailoring communication meets a patient's individual needs and promotes comprehensive understanding and participation in health goals. Choice *A* is incorrect as alternative communication formats can be utilized via online delivery or face-to-face, depending on the patient's preferences and healthcare needs. Choice *C* is incorrect as the patient should be encouraged to fully interact with the healthcare team to the utmost of their capabilities, and a representative should be selected by the patient or by the court if the patient is unable to do so. Choice *D* is incorrect; translation services may be used for sensory deficit patients—such as sign language services or foreign

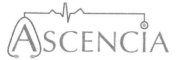

language interpretation—which may be required in addition to alternative communication due to sensory impairment needs.

26. C: The answer is Choice *C.* In effective conflict management, the nurse manager would address the conflict as early as possible, listen to both parties in a nonjudgmental manner, and clarify the issue to determine a goal and seek resolution.

27. B: The correct answer is Choice *B*, as oxycodone is a narcotic and should be discarded in the controlled waste receptacle. Regulated medical waste, sinks, and sharps containers are not approved locations for medication disposal.

28. C: Choice *C* is correct, as subjective data is qualitative and based on the patient's own perception and description of the pain. Choices *A* and *D* both describe data that may be perceived, measured, and analyzed. Choice *B* is not a label used to describe patient data.

29. A: The correct answer is Choice *A* as empathy is the state of showing that another's feelings and emotions are understood and shared. Choice *B* is incorrect as implicit biases are stereotypes and preconceived notions that are not yet known or explored. Choice *C* is not correct as sympathy is a feeling of sorrow for someone else's distress; it is not understanding the other's feelings. Choice *D* is not correct as active listening is a process that involves receiving the patient's message, interpreting the meaning, and responding to reflect the speaker's needs.

30. D: The answer is Choice *D.* In team nursing, nurses work together collaboratively. The team nursing model is beneficial for novice staff. A skilled nurse is the team leader, who uses leadership skills and must communicate effectively. Total patient care delivery is when one nurse is assigned to a group of patients during the shift. In the primary care model, one nurse is accountable for the care delivered. The functional nursing care model is the framework in which tasks are assigned by a charge nurse.

31. C: Nursing-Sensitive Indicators (NSIs) are crucial for monitoring and improving the quality of nursing care, assessing its impact on patient outcomes, and making data-driven decisions to enhance nursing practice. Although cost-effectiveness may be a consideration, NSIs primarily focus on patient care quality and safety, and therefore Choice *A* is incorrect. Choice *B* is incorrect because marketing efforts are not the primary purpose of NSIs. Choice *D* is not accurate, as NSIs are primarily concerned with assessing and improving nursing care and its impact on patient outcomes, not identifying new medical treatments.

32. D: The correct answer is Choice *D* as the formal request of medical records via organizational policy is the appropriate avenue to receive physical printouts of the medical record. Due to legalities, Choices *A*, *B*, and *C* must not print out anything from the chart but instead direct the patient to the medical records department per policy.

33. C: The answer is Choice *C*, as financial stewardship involves managing resources and eliminating unnecessary costs, including excessive overtime. Nursing leaders work within a budget that includes staff productive working hours. Nurses can be financial stewards by working within scheduled hours and not creating the need for overtime.

34. B: The correct answer is Choice *B*; type I diabetes requires insulin administration to maintain an euglycemic state since insulin production is insufficient or completely absent. Choices *A*, *C*, and *D* are all attributes of type II diabetes.

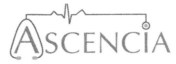

35. B: The correct answer is Choice *B*, as the nurse should FIRST wash the exposure site thoroughly with soap and water IMMEDIATELY. Next, he should notify the charge nurse and receive medical attention. A safety report should be filed, although this would not take priority.

36. B: Choice *B* is the correct answer as this is targeted at all staff within the organization and encourages self-reflection to address understanding one's own responsibility in preventing implicit bias. Choice *A* is incorrect as training should be ongoing, not a one-time class. Choice *C* is incorrect because it only provides training to bedside staff; true cultural change must include all staff and providers. Choice *D* is incorrect because training should focus on the micro and macro aspects of racial biases.

37. A: The Academy of Medical-Surgical Nurses (AMSN) Scope and Standards of Practice emphasizes the nursing role in advocating for the patient's well-being by providing interventions that are not only evidence-based but also aligned with the patient's preferences and wishes. It underscores the importance of patient-centered care, respecting the patient's autonomy, choices, and values. Choice *B* is incorrect because implementing interventions solely based on clinical evidence does not fully capture the patient-centered approach highlighted in the standards, which considers both evidence-based care and the patient's preferences. Choice *C* is incorrect because prioritizing the nurse's recommendations over the patient's choices contradicts the patient-centered approach advocated in the standards, which places the patient's wishes at the forefront. Choice *D* is incorrect because fostering a one-sided approach to patient care does not align with the collaborative and patient-centered approach promoted by the AMSN Scope and Standards of Practice.

38. C: The correct answer is Choice *C*; aspiration can present itself shortly after eating. This is evaluated by having the patient speak after eating. If there is any sign of dyspnea, the test is immediately aborted. Choice *A* is not appropriate until the patient has been fully evaluated for safety with swallowing. Choice *B*, a barium swallow study would be ordered after signs of aspiration, which still needs to be fully assessed for this patient. Choice *D* would not be anticipated until diagnostic testing, such as a barium study, is completed and indicates that further evaluation is needed.

39. A: The correct answer is Choice *A*. Behaviors suspicious for drug diversion include retrieving medication from the automated dispensing cabinet more than 30 minutes prior to the administration time, delaying waste documentation, not using appropriate dose sizes, and arriving early or staying late.

40. D: Choice *D* is correct, as an outcome that is not fully met may need an additional treatment to increase the probability that the patient will respond to current interventions that are having some, but not all, positive effects in meeting outcomes. Choice *A* is not correct, as treatment is aimed at improving the patient to their baseline or greater; this would mean that the current treatment has been effective. Choice *B* is not correct because the current treatment needs to be partially effective and not ineffective. Choice *C* is not correct, as an adjuvant or additive treatment makes the current treatment stronger; the current treatment should be discontinued if the patient cannot tolerate it.

41. A: The correct answer is Choice *A*, as advocacy is the support of a certain nursing issue that affects patient care. Autonomy and self-determination refer to the ability to make one's own choices. Opposition is the resistance to a certain policy.

42. A: The correct answer is Choice *A*. The patient's immediate safety should be addressed first. Strapping the patient to the bed with a sheet is considered a restraint because it restricts freedom of movement. A safety report should be filed and the nurse manager should be notified. However, the patient's safety takes precedence. Assessing the patient's cognition is appropriate as ongoing care, but would not address the immediate need of the patient.

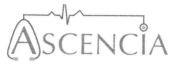

43. C: The correct answer is Choice *C*; interdisciplinary rounds that include the patient uphold information sharing and provide the patient with an opportunity to be updated on the care plan and ask questions. Family presence is encouraged at the patient's discretion. Choice *A* is inappropriate; discharge planning should occur as soon as possible in the patient's stay, and this answer choice does not support patient participation and autonomy. Choice *B* is not correct because this takes the interdisciplinary approach away from the patient's bedside and does not allow the patient to ask questions directly to the care team. Choice *D* is incorrect because a nursing bedside report provides a similar effect on the patient's participation with care as does interdisciplinary rounding by facilitating patient-centered communication.

44. B: The answer is Choice *B*. The logistics branch of the hospital incident command system (HCIS) directs resources, including equipment, supplies, and workers, so the healthcare system may effectively accomplish the work during the disaster. The other selections have a different role. The liaison officer speaks with external organizations and other emergency response partners. The public information officer coordinates the methods for dispersal of communication, and the security and safety officer communicates with law enforcement.

45. A: The correct answer is Choice *A*. A sign of vancomycin toxicity is ototoxicity, a ringing or humming in the ears. The nurse should stop the medication to prevent further patient injury. The other choices are not the best responses: Administering an antibiotic will likely decrease the patient's temperature, losartan's peak effect occurs 1–2 hours after intake, and the production of diarrhea after lactulose is expected.

46. D: The correct answer is Choice *D*; food should be chewed thoroughly prior to swallowing. Choice *A* is incorrect because the cuff should be deflated, not inflated, so that swallowing is not impeded. Choice *B* is not correct; liquids should be thickened to increase resistance to flow. Thin liquids can easily flow into the airway. Choice *C* is incorrect as small bites are easier to manage than larger bites when implementing swallowing precautions.

47. C: Burnout is characterized by emotional exhaustion, depersonalization (cynical or negative attitudes toward work and patients), and reduced personal accomplishment. It often results from prolonged exposure to chronic workplace stress and can significantly impact the well-being and job performance of healthcare professionals. Choice *A* is incorrect because moral distress and moral injuries are related to ethical dilemmas and the misalignment of personal values with workplace actions but do not include the specific dimensions of burnout. Choice *B* is incorrect because compassion fatigue refers to emotional exhaustion and reduced compassion but does not typically involve depersonalization or reduced personal accomplishment as seen in burnout. Choice *D* is incorrect because job dissatisfaction is a broader concept that may result from various workplace factors and does not specifically capture the multifaceted nature of burnout.

48. B: The correct answer is Choice *B*, as this enhances safe medication administration two-fold, with a current medication index as well as programmed safe limits. All IV pumps, regardless of "smart" functions, are intended to provide controlled delivery of the medication that is referenced in Choice *A*. The lock-out function of Choice *C* does enhance safety; however, it is not the BEST choice to support medication administration safety. Choice *D* reduces desensitization to alarms but does not alter medication administration safety.

49. B: The correct answer is Choice *B*. The patient's pills should be kept out of reach but not stored in the bathroom where there is a high level of humidity.

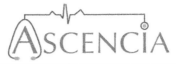

50. A: The correct answer is Choice A. Since many Hispanic families center their family time around food, being able to have home-cooked food that he is familiar with may encourage appetite. Choice B does not provide the patient with choices that he is familiar with or has stated that he enjoys. Being non-compliant with the diet would indicate the patient is eating something that is restricted, which is not the case suggested by Choice C. Choice D may provide the patient with an option that he would find more pleasing; however, it does not address the social aspect of wanting a connection to home.

51. B: The correct answer is Choice B. The nurse should develop the habit of always logging out of charting systems prior to leaving the work station. While most systems have a timed logout, the nurse should not allow ANY time that PHI is readily accessible to anyone that walks by. This is important for protecting patient privacy and for preventing an open opportunity for a hacker. Sharing a patient's name over text and unencrypted emails can lead to major cybersecurity risks. Computer software updates are critical in preventing malware. While most facilities require the IT department to be involved in computer updates, the nurse should not reschedule a scheduled update time. The IT department should be promptly notified. Lastly, the nurse should not use common passwords that are used for other logins. Passwords with birthdates/names or common words are at risk for hacking. Passwords should also be changed every six months.

52. C: The answer is Choice C, as this nurse is describing her own nursing philosophy. Nursing philosophy is a set of intrinsic values that guides the practice of the nurse. These values often encompass personal experiences and beliefs about the nursing profession. Caring and ethics are common themes in a philosophy statement. Clinical judgment is the skill of making an inference about a patient's needs.

53. A: Choice A is correct, as the goal is to provide comprehensive, collaborative care with open communication and alignment with multiple discipline-led interventions to meet outcomes. Choice B is incorrect, as the focus should be on a holistic approach, not just disease driven, and also managing signs and symptoms as well as integrating specialty care, such as restorative care, physical therapy, and dietary management. Choice C is incorrect, as communication should never be kept from the patient or caretaker. Patient-centered care advocates for the patient being a contributing member to the healthcare team. Choice D is incorrect, as specialty departments must actively communicate within their own service and the entire care team to share pertinent information related to the patient's care plan and moving toward meeting the patient's goals.

54. A: Choice A is correct as, ideally, any advance directives should be completed and on file prior to an emergency. Choice B is incorrect as this depicts a certain event that may have risks; by this point, advance directives should have already been addressed. Choice C is incorrect because during an emergency, the patient may not have full capacity to give a reasonable request or may not be responsive. Choice D is incorrect; advance directives are most effective when patient wishes are discussed and decided prior to a major life event.

55. D: Emotional workplace safety aims to ensure the psychological and emotional well-being of healthcare professionals by fostering a supportive workplace culture where staff members feel comfortable expressing their opinions and concerns without fear of reprisal or judgment. This goal is crucial because it helps create an environment where healthcare professionals can effectively cope with the challenges they encounter, such as stressful shifts, conflicts, and adaptability requirements. It promotes a sense of belonging, mutual support, and open communication, ultimately enhancing job satisfaction and overall quality of care. Choice A misrepresents emotional workplace safety by suggesting that it seeks to eliminate all workplace challenges, which is not feasible. Choice B focuses on physical well-being, neglecting the critical aspect of emotional and psychological support. Choice C

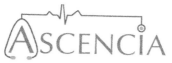

oversimplifies the concept by reducing it to the freedom to express opinions without acknowledging the broader goals and benefits of emotional workplace safety.

56. B: The correct answer is Choice B; lobster is a shellfish and does not have scales or fins, and thus is not allowed. Choices A, C, and D are allowed per Jewish law.

57. B: The correct answer is Choice B. Patients are at risk of medication error when there is lack of direction indicating the proper rate of IV push medication administration. Following the physician order, looking in an institution-approved drug reference guide, or reviewing instructions on the medication administration record are ways the nurse can obtain the proper rate. Preparing medication away from the bedside can be a risk of harm, especially when not labeling the syringe. Other risks include medication that is transferred from one place to another or diluted.

58. B: The correct answer is Choice B; the gold standard for administering TPN is a central line, such as a PICC, as TPN is highly caustic to the inner lumen of peripheral vasculature and has a significantly increased risk for thromboembolism. A mid-line, Choice A, and IV, Choice B, would not be appropriate as they deliver directly to the periphery, increasing the risk of phlebitis. These lines do not extend to the central vena cava where the vessels are larger and allow for more turbulent dispersion of the TPN fluid. A PEG is a type of gastronomy tube. TPN is not delivered via the vascular system, not the gastrointestinal system.

59. C: The correct answer is Choice C. The nurse would be concerned about signs of human trafficking. The patient should be spoken to in privacy, without the potential controller being present. Because the patient speaks little English, a translator should be scheduled. The nurse should perform a comprehensive assessment, observing any signs of physical abuse. Open-ended questions allow the victim the opportunity to describe her situation.

60. B: The correct answer is Choice B. Missing or unclear documentation is a hazard as documentation is required to appropriately guide effective patient care. Choice A is incorrect as this does not increase access to health data. Choice C is incorrect as treatment decisions will not be guided by the whole clinical picture. Choice D is incorrect as clinicians will spend increased time seeking patient data, not less.

61. C: The correct answer is Choice C. Polypharmacy, defined as taking multiple medications, may lead to additional side effects that would not occur if the drugs were given separately. This can lead to a prescribing cascade.

62. D: Choice D is correct, as a dependent nursing intervention must be initiated by an order from a medical practitioner. Choices A and C describe an interdependent nursing intervention that is collaborative and reliant upon another discipline to complete. Independent nursing interventions, described in Choice B, are those that can be instituted and performed by the nurse without an order or direction from another and are within the nurse's scope of practice.

63. A: The answer is Choice A. In the ADKAR change model (Awareness, Desire, Knowledge, Ability, Reinforcement), the nurse manager would use strategies that involve the final step in the process, Reinforcement. These include providing positive reinforcement and feedback, as well as celebrating successes. Creating awareness occurs in the first step. Piloting a trial is accomplished in the Ability step, and providing in-service training occurs in the Knowledge step.

64. C: The correct answer is Choice C, as nasogastric tubes may become dislodged, resulting in a high risk of fluid being delivered into the lungs. Choice A is not likely as feeding pumps deliver formula at a set rate over time. Formula leaking from the tube is unlikely to be a cause, as in Choice B. The patient, not

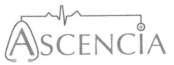

the device, is the nurse's priority while troubleshooting an alarm. Choice *D* may be considered AFTER the patient is assessed.

65. C: The correct answer is Choice *C*; the patient's beliefs should not be assumed. There are varying levels of religious practices that people follow, and it is best practice to ask the patient what their preference is. Choice *A* is not correct because the nurse is overstepping boundaries in the patient-nurse relationship by fixing what is a perceived issue without checking with the patient. Choice *B* is not correct because when traditional Jewish culture is adhered to, meat and dairy are not eaten together. Choice *D* is not correct because the nurse has identified a potential issue with the patient's order based on their stated religion. The patient should be consulted first on whether the order is correct to ensure that the patient's beliefs and practices are upheld.

66. D: The correct answer is Choice *D*. A urinary output of less than 30mL/hr could be a sign of sepsis. Other signs include cognitive changes, respiratory rate of more than 20 breaths/minute, temperature of greater than 101 °F/38.3 °C or less than 96.8 °F/36 °C, edema, and systolic blood pressure <90 mm Hg.

67. A: The correct answer is Choice *A*. The nurse is ultimately accountable for the task completion. The nursing assistant also has accountability for the task that was delegated to them. The other selections are incorrect. The nurse is responsible for determining patient needs. The institution or state Nurse Practice Act determines the nursing responsibilities that can be delegated. The nursing assistant does not have to accept the task if she is not able to perform it.

68. C: Choice *C* is correct, as role clarification allows the team to coordinate care quickly and effectively in response to emergent situations. Choice *A* is incorrect, as role clarification may not directly affect the amount of reporting that occurs but may make the reporting more effective by leading team members to respond more succinctly to requests. Choice *B* is not correct, as not all team members may be able to round concurrently, but role establishment can allow an appointed leader to relay information to the patient. Choice *D* is not correct, as roles should be established as a level team; hierarchical teams have been found to be unconducive to data sharing and collaboration.

69. D: The correct answer is Choice *D*. The nurse is surprised that she received an order for warfarin and must contact the ordering provider to inquire about the purpose of the drug. This fulfills medication administration safety and meets the right indication and the right patient. The nurse can implement all the actions described, but the priority is the patient's immediate safety.

70. D: The correct answer is Choice *D*; a patient who has not passed a bedside swallow study should be evaluated via a barium swallow study before being allowed to try to intake any other food by mouth. The patient should be further evaluated before repeating the study the next day or allowing the food that the patient was able to swallow; therefore, Choices *A* and *B* are incorrect. At this time, the patient shows no indications that the swallowing issue is long-term, so Choice *C*, a G-tube, is not appropriate.

71. C: The correct answer is Choice *C*; since the first step of process improvement is the identification of the issue, the nurse informaticist would start by analyzing the issue. Choices *A* and *D* both apply a solution to the problem that occurs after the problem is identified. Choice *B* would occur last, after the change has been implemented and trialed for a determined amount of time.

72. B: The correct answer is Choice *B*; a chest x-ray should be ordered with the image indicating that the NG tube is 10 centimeters past the gastroesophageal junction and the tip is visualized below the left hemi diaphragm. The pH of gastric aspirate may be tested for acidity as a way to verify placement; however, the result should be ≤ 5.5, not > as Choice *A* indicates. Choice *C* is incorrect as although this is used to check for placement, it is not the gold standard for initially verifying placement. A newly placed

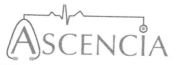

NG tube must always be verified prior to first use to prevent aspiration. Choice *D* is incorrect as the tube may be coiled within the trachea, esophagus, or pharynx and not cause symptoms.

73. A: The answer is Choice *A*. During the mitigation phase, the community risks are assessed and resources are identified. The goal is to lessen harm as much as possible. The second phase is preparedness, when the plan details are determined. The other two options are not applicable to the question.

74. C: The correct answer is Choice *C*. A high-alert medication is defined as a medication that requires a heightened alert because the drug can potentially cause significant patient harm when used in error. All of the options are correct statements about heparin, but the best response is Choice *C*.

75. B: Choice *B* is correct, as the nursing process is fluid and can move along the elements to quickly adapt to a patient's needs. Choice *A* is incorrect because the treatment may not be effective, and continuing may be futile; the treatment plan should be revisited for other interventions and options. Choice *C* is not correct, as it may just mean that the intervention was not effective and another treatment should be considered. Not meeting all outcomes is, at times, expected. The care plan would not be discontinued as suggested in Choice *D*; it would be revisited and updated to adjust the outcomes or incorporate new interventions.

76. B: In this scenario, the nurse should report the incident to their immediate supervisor or charge nurse. This is the appropriate action to take when observing a colleague completing a procedure outside their authorized scope of practice to ensure patient safety and maintain professional standards. Choice *A* is incorrect, as it may lead to a potentially confrontational or unproductive situation. If the situation has the potential to bring harm to the patient, the nurse should intervene in an appropriate manner. Confronting the colleague at the bedside can create both conflict and a barrier of mistrust with the patient. Choice *C* is not an appropriate response because it involves a potential breach of professional boundaries and patient safety. Choice *D* may not be within the nurse's scope of practice, nor does it address the ethical concern.

77. D: The correct answer is Choice *D*, as visual cues provide an additional reminder to critical alerts and enhance patient safety. Choices *A* and *B* add additional steps and decrease efficiency. These are not attributes that contribute to improving patient safety. Hard stops do not allow a user to perform an action that has a high potential for an adverse reaction. Choice *C* cancels the purpose of this safety feature.

78. B: The answer is Choice *B*. In order to increase job engagement and retention, the nurse manager can ask a newer nurse to be involved in a work environment committee, as part of shared governance. Obligatory certification or education and reprimanding staff are not ways to increase retention.

79. C: The correct answer is Choice *C*. The most effective way to mitigate complaints is to ensure that the patient understands the capabilities of the care team in achieving the goals of the care plan as well as to establish whether the patient's expectations are reasonable. Choice *A* is not correct as the provider should not provide false hope or promises that are outside of their control. Choice *B* is incorrect as it is unethical and against most organizations' policies to provide a different level of care based on a patient's social status. Choice *D* is incorrect as this establishes a standard that all complaints be resolved through reward and can lead to further complications.

80. A: Choice *A* is correct, as the priority interventions should follow the fundamentals of maintaining the airway, breathing, and circulation. Supplemental oxygen improves myocardial oxygenation levels to decrease the onset of cardiac ischemia. Choices *B* and *C* are incorrect, as these do not immediately

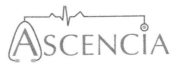

relieve the nursing diagnosis of acute pain. Choice *D* is not correct, as it does not relate to either the medical or nursing diagnosis.

81. B: The correct answer is Choice *B*. In a culture of safety, active communication and speaking up is important to providing timely feedback. The nurse can promote teamwork by addressing the safety concern first with her coworker and teaching her the correct technique. Because this issue is a near-miss of a needlestick injury, the situation should be reported in an internal safety report because there may be a need for further education on the device use.

82. A: The correct answer is Choice *A*; any patient with new onset facial drooping should be evaluated for signs and symptoms of a stroke. Spastic movements, Choice *B*, are a sign of Parkinson's disease. Throat pain and dry throat are common side effects related to medications used to treat neurological disorders, so Choice *C* is incorrect. A sudden headache, not chest pain as in Choice *D*, may be a symptom of a stroke.

83. B: Choice *B* is correct, as an assessment guides the next steps of the nursing process. Choices *A*, *C*, and *D* are completed in the following order after the assessment: diagnosis, planning, and implementation.

84. D: The correct answer is Choice *D*, as verifying an artificial airway via chest x-ray is the best practice. Choices *A*, *B*, and *C* are used to check for proper placement of a nasogastric tube, not an oropharyngeal tube.

85. B: The correct answer is Choice *B*. The mentor and mentee enter a long-term professional relationship that enhances growth and development. The mentor provides a supportive environment so that the mentee can share difficult encounters. Assessing the nurse's competence and teaching are the roles of a preceptor, which is a short-term relationship. A coach encourages self-assessment and reflection.

86. C: The correct answer is Choice *C*, as towel racks are not meant to support the patient's weight and could result in a fall. Grab bars should be installed to assist the patient to sit from a standing position so that the patient does not lose balance. The other choices do not require further follow-up.

87. B: The correct answer is Choice *B*. Nurses should have limited access to high-alert medications. Other strategies to reduce medication risk and patient harm include standardizing medication preparation, ensuring access to drug information, and affixing cautionary labels.

88. B: The correct answer is Choice *B* as corn tortillas are gluten-free. Choice *A* is incorrect because a brioche roll is made with wheat. Barley is a gluten-containing grain, making Choice *C* incorrect. Choice *D* is incorrect; while oats are gluten-free, they are often contaminated with wheat products as the FDA only requires that food packaged as oats contain less than 20 parts per million of gluten overall.

89. C: Patients have the responsibility to provide accurate and complete medical information to their healthcare providers, including details about their medical history, current medications, allergies, and any relevant health conditions. This information is crucial in order for healthcare providers to make informed decisions about patient care and treatment. Choices *A*, *B*, and *D* are incorrect because they are actually patient rights, not responsibilities.

90. D: The correct answer is Choice *D*. The patient is diagnosed with influenza, which requires droplet and contact precautions. The daughter will need to wear a gown, goggles, a mask, and gloves. The droplets often suspend and fall within three feet.

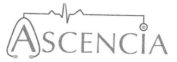

91. D: The correct answer is Choice *D*. A sentinel event causes permanent harm or injury that is not the result of the disease process itself. In this case, the patient fell and sustained a subdural hematoma. Although the patient may have experienced an adverse event or a side effect from the medication, the cause of falling is not indicated. A root cause analysis may determine that the fall was the result of receiving the medication.

92. C: Choice *C* is correct, as the nursing diagnosis is obtained from a list published by NANDA International and is a diagnosis that describes the effects of a medical diagnosis. Choice *A* is incorrect because making a medical diagnosis is outside the scope of practice of a nurse. Choice *B* is incorrect because the nursing diagnosis is used to understand the body's response to the disease process. Choice *D* is incorrect because the primary treatment of the patient is guided by the medical diagnosis.

93. D: The answer is Choice *D*. Compromising is often used when a quick solution is required, but it does not thoroughly explore the problem. Both parties must give up a conviction in order to accomplish the task at hand. In this instance, the nurse will help and the nursing assistant must answer call lights. Accommodating refers to when the relationship is put aside, no matter the outcome of the conflict. Collaborating occurs when both people work together towards the goal with a desire to protect the relationship. Competing occurs when the goals of both parties are sought, no matter the cost of the relationship.

94. B: The Nursing Code of Ethics places a central emphasis on safeguarding patient autonomy and advocating for their best interests. Nurses are entrusted with the responsibility of ensuring that patients' best interests are paramount in all healthcare decisions and actions, promoting informed consent, and facilitating open and honest communication between patients and healthcare teams. This aligns with the core principle of patient advocacy in nursing ethics. Choice *A* is incorrect because it focuses on the financial aspect of healthcare institutions, which is not the primary focus of nursing ethics. Choice *C* is incorrect because it emphasizes expediting procedures to minimize costs, which may not necessarily align with patient-centered care. Choice *D* is incorrect because it prioritizes healthcare providers' convenience and comfort, which is not a primary focus in nursing ethics, where the patient's well-being is paramount.

95. A: The correct answer is Choice *A*. Moral disengagement occurs when there is a disassociation of ethical standards from a certain situation without feeling remorse. The principle of nonmaleficence is defined as doing no harm by selecting interventions that achieve the best outcome. An intentional tort is described as deliberately committing wrongdoing. Paternalism refers to making decisions for a patient without their consent, such as hiding a diagnosis or treatment option.

96. D: The correct answer is Choice *D*; unless not culturally acceptable, maintaining eye contact that is natural and facing the patient shows respect and is an active listening stance. Choice *A* assumes that the patient does not speak English based on documented race. Choice *B* is an intimidating pose that may make the patient feel uncomfortable and unable to establish trust with the provider. Choice *C* is incorrect as interrupting can make the patient feel like they are not being listened to and does not support patient-centered care.

97. C: The correct answer is Choice *C*, as any malfunctioning equipment, especially devices used with patients, should be immediately removed from service and tagged according to agency policy. Choice *A* may cause harm to the patient. By placing it in the supply closet without any indication that the device is not working properly, another healthcare member might use it with a patient; therefore, Choice *B* is not appropriate. Healthcare staff should not take it upon themselves to throw away equipment as suggested in Choice *D*. The equipment may be repaired or under warranty.

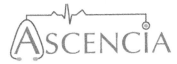

98. D: Choice *D* is the correct answer, as the patient should first be consulted regarding their own health history, unless the patient has a cognitive disorder or is a poor historian. Choices *A*, *B*, and *C* are all secondary sources for the patient's history.

99. C: The correct answer is Choice *C*. When the nurse finds out that the patient cannot afford her medications, the nurse alerts the interdisciplinary team because the patient's wound may not heal if she does not take the full dose of antibiotics as prescribed. The other options are not correct. Generic drugs are often cheaper than brand-name drugs. The insurance company alerts the patient about the copay required. The antibiotic would not necessarily be discontinued, unless the patient has received the full dose.

100. A: Choice *A* is correct, as the outcome described does not have a time frame added and therefore does not meet all elements of a SMART goal. Choice *B* is incorrect, as the goal has a measurable element of the oxygen saturation. Choices *C* and *D* are incorrect, as the goal specifies measures that are conducive to treating the primary issue of shortness of breath.

101. B: The answer is Choice *B*, as nursing peer review is the process by which nurses of the same professional position and clinical expertise evaluate another nurse to enhance self-regulation and increase accountability. The other three options do not pertain to the situation. Peer evaluation is used as part of nursing performance evaluations.

102. C: The correct answer is Choice *C*, as Meaningful Use was established by the U.S. government to set minimum standards for the use of the electronic health record. Choice *A*, Health Insurance Portability and Accountability Act (HIPAA), is a federal law that enforces the protection of private health information. Choice *B* is a healthcare initiative that supports community and individual health with data-driven national objectives. Choice *D*, Equitable Long-Term Recovery and Resilience, is a federal agency cooperative aimed at improving the health of individuals and communities across the nation.

103. D: The answer is Choice *D*. Competencies are a group of abilities needed for the nurse to accomplish his role, established on knowledge, skills, and attitude. Competence is a distinct term meaning the success at carrying out a professional responsibility. Aptitude is a person's natural ability, and capability is the potential to accomplish a task.

104. C: Choice *C* is correct, as effective communication and collaboration within the interdisciplinary team have been shown to have a positive effect on patient outcomes. Choice *A* is incorrect, as the goal is not to decrease interruptions but to increase positive interactions and teamwork. Choice *B* is incorrect, as continuous, not intermittent, critical thinking should drive patient care. Choice *D* is incorrect, as the patient's disease process will determine the level of acuity.

105. D: The correct answer is Choice *D*, as the nurse prefers the visual learning style. A visual learner likes to draw, uses color codes, and often highlights text as a way to remember information. An auditory learner prefers to listen. A kinesthetic learner will learn by doing. A learner who likes reading often prefers reading text or rewriting their notes.

106. B: The correct answer is Choice *B*; convenience foods often lack the needed macro and micro nutrients for a healthy diet. Choices *A*, *C*, and *D* do not put the patient at a higher risk for food resource limitations.

107. C: The answer is Choice *C*, as the nurse manager serves as the liaison between the staff nurse and upper nursing leadership team and runs the daily operations of the nursing unit. The director of nursing oversees multiple medical-surgical nursing units. The charge nurse directs and coordinates workflow during the shift. The chief nursing officer establishes the nursing strategic plan.

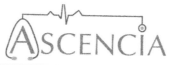

108. A: The correct answer is Choice *A*, as antimicrobials can disturb the gut microbiome. Administering foods high in probiotics, including kefir, yogurt, kombucha, sauerkraut, and tempeh, helps to reestablish the beneficial microbes and prevent diarrhea. Probiotic supplements are also a good option.

109. A: The correct answer is Choice *A*; blood sugar levels may fluctuate significantly when TPN is initially started. This requires frequent finger stick blood sugar checks, and pharmacies may add insulin to the formula to prevent hyperglycemic events. Choice *C* is not as critical to check in the first 72 hours, although TPN may cause diarrhea due to the high glucose content and effects on insulin release, potentially leading to hypokalemia. Hyper- or hyponatremia is not a significant risk with TPN administration, so Choice *B* is incorrect. Elevated white blood cells can indicate an infection, which is a significant risk with TPN administration, but this is monitored closely throughout TPN administration, so Choice *D* is incorrect.

110. B: The answer is Choice *B*. The triaging of patients occurs by classification. The most emergent patients are those with life-threatening injuries and immediate needs, including chest pain, severe respiratory distress, acute neurological conditions, and amputation. An urgent patient sustains non-life-threatening injuries, like open fractures. Minor lacerations and an ankle sprain are not urgent.

111. B: The correct answer is Choice *B*. The nurse responsible for the preoperative nursing assessment, handling certain surgical instruments, and providing hemostasis is the registered nurse first assistant (RNFA). The registered nurse circulator performs a preoperative nursing assessment, serves as the patient advocate, and oversees the surgical activities. The surgical scrub nurse maintains and safeguards the sterile field. They work directly with the surgeon by handing surgical instruments. The vascular access nurse is responsible for maintaining central lines.

112. B: The answer is Choice *B*. With a democratic leadership style, staff input is a factor in decision-making. An autocratic style occurs when a leader makes decisions without staff participation. Laissez-faire involves staff making independent decisions, and a transformational style applies when leaders encourage staff to work towards a greater vision.

113. C: The correct answer is Choice *C* as pausing the pump stops the medication delivery and silences the alarm briefly while the issue can be safely discovered and resolved. Choice *A* should occur after the pump is paused. Choice *B* should be avoided without further evidence of the patient manipulating the pump as this is unnecessarily accusatory. Choice *D* is one of the most common causes of IV pump alarms; however, it is best practice to first pause the pump.

114. A: The correct answer is Choice *A*; heart failure exacerbation is primarily caused by fluid retention. Sodium causes the body to retain water, leading to fluid volume overload and strain on the heart muscle. Choice *B* is incorrect; it may be a modifiable factor to reduce the risk for hypertension, but it is unlikely that occasional alcohol use will exacerbate heart failure. Choices *C* and *D* are interventions to prevent or treat fluid volume overload, not causes of it.

115. C: The correct answer is Choice *C*. Nitroglycerin is considered hazardous pharmaceutical waste. Medications are disposed of in their proper pharmaceutical waste bin and not down the toilet or sink.

116. C: Choice *C* is correct, as the blood loss is something that can be measured and has a specific numeric value. Choices *A*, *B*, and *D* are all subjective data based on the patient's experience, opinions, and feelings.

117. A: The answer is Choice *A*. The nurse manager serves as an advocate when stressful events occur, such as a patient death or crisis. They create a supportive environment, listen, remain objective and calm, debrief, and offer compassion.

Answer Explanations #1

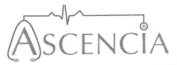

118. A: The correct answer is Choice *A*; intake of fortified dairy is the main source of calciferol (vitamin D), as it is not found naturally in many foods. High sources of magnesium, Choice *B*, are found in nuts, seeds, legumes, and dark leafy greens, not in dairy. Choice *C* is provided by dairy, but it is also provided in sufficient amounts in other foods such as eggs, lean meats, fruits, and vegetables. Choice *D*, *ascorbic acid* (vitamin C), is provided in high quantities via citrus fruits.

119. A: The correct answer is Choice *A*, as watchdog data collection is a consultative service that analyzes patient care areas to seek areas for improvement and identify deficits in standards of care. Choice *B* is incorrect as patient surveys are distributed by an organization's advocacy department or by publicly reporting bodies, such as HCAHPS, and are not part of the watchdog's tasks. Choice *C* is incorrect as watchdog data collection is not aimed at staff but at improving systems to enhance patient care. Choice *D* is incorrect as quality reviews are typically completed by a department that focuses on patient care from the lens of quality, safety, and value or by accrediting bodies during inspections.

120. A: The answer is Choice *A*. A systematic process involving assessment, planning, implementation, and evaluation refers to the nursing process. The other statements about clinical judgment are correct.

121. A: Choice *A* is correct, as it is data that is important for the care team to readily know upon entering a patient's room in order to keep the patient safe and free from harm. Choice *B* is not correct, as this may be hurtful or embarrassing to the patient and can potentially harm the trust between the patient and care team. Choice *C* does not impact the patient's care and is not appropriate to put in a visible place. Choice *D* is incorrect, as it is protected health information and publishing it publicly would violate HIPAA.

122. C: The correct answer is Choice *C*. Although all these actions are part of precepting, the most important role is to assess the preceptee's competence and ability to provide safe patient care.

123. D: The correct answer is Choice *D*; while kidney dysfunction filters out the metabolites formed from protein breakdown, the breakdown of protein is caused by the release of digestive enzymes by the pancreas to the digestive system. Choices *A*, *B*, and *C* are all functions of the renal system.

124. C: The correct answer is Choice *C*; through being a subject matter expert and providing education to colleagues with a wide-scale audience, the nurse has achieved the stated goals. Choices *A* and *B* are incorrect because they increase the nurse's own education, not others. Choice *D* is incorrect because it aims to improve patient safety through the development of policy, not education.

125. C: Choice *C* is correct as hospice care is offered when all curative measures have been exhausted and the patient's condition is declining. Choice *A* is incorrect because it is describing palliative care, not hospice. Choice *B* is incorrect because hospice care is designed for end-of-life care, whereas palliative care incorporates curative measures. Choice *D* is incorrect as there are strict criteria for both palliative and hospice care.

Practice Test #2

1. What is the primary purpose of reviewing existing literature and studies related to a chosen research topic before initiating a clinical research study?
   a. To identify potential research participants for the study
   b. To build a foundation of knowledge and understand the current state of knowledge on the topic
   c. To generate hypotheses for the research study
   d. To collect data from previous research to support the study's findings

2. What is a best practice strategy to decrease patient complaints?
   a. Apply a retroactive stance when addressing concerns
   b. Train front-line staff on passive listening
   c. Promote empathic and active listening
   d. Form a specialized team that provides service recovery for all concerns prior to escalation

3. A newly licensed nurse is hired to work on a medical-surgical nursing unit. She understands that there will be an orientation process where she will meet with nurse educators and also be assigned a preceptor for several weeks. She understands that the purpose of orientation is best explained as a time period for:
   a. testing and validating the content that she learned in her nursing program.
   b. developing knowledge and competence in her clinical setting to best care for patients.
   c. developing skills so that she will not need to have any accountability while learning.
   d. learning everything she needs to know in order to transition into her role seamlessly.

4. A 46-year-old female is readmitted to the medical-surgical unit after experiencing a foul odor from her surgical incision. The nurse gathers supplies to take a wound culture and apply a clean dressing. The nurse is concerned that the patient has a surgical site infection, most related to which factor?
   a. The patient has a body mass index (BMI) of 24.
   b. The patient received a warming blanket prior to surgery.
   c. Supplemental oxygen was delivered during surgery.
   d. The length of surgery was longer than expected.

5. Which of the following statements are true regarding durable power of attorney?
   a. It allows a designated agent to make healthcare decisions on behalf of the patient.
   b. It is not legally binding.
   c. It always gives authority to the next of kin.
   d. The designated agent makes financial decisions if the patient is incapacitated.

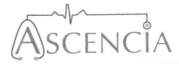

6. A 78-year-old female is admitted to the nursing unit with bilateral pneumonia. The nurse is performing a physical assessment and notes that the patient has erythema at the postauricular region of the ear. The patient reports soreness. The nurse knows that the skin integrity of the patient is compromised due to the nasal cannula medical device. Which intervention can the nurse use to alleviate further harm?

    a. A thin layer of water-based lubricant applied to the reddened area
    b. Removal of the nasal cannula and placement of a continuous pulse oximeter on the patient
    c. Tightening of the nasal cannula tubing to prevent excess rubbing from loose tubing
    d. Placement of a hydrocolloid dressing between the device and the injured skin

7. A nurse is preparing to provide a hand-off report to the oncoming nurse. What best practice has been identified to support patient-centered care and safety in medical-surgical units?

    a. Standardized electronic report
    b. Bedside report
    c. SBAR
    d. Interdisciplinary rounding

8. A 56-year-old male patient is transferred from the medical-surgical nursing unit to the operating room for a small bowel resection due to an obstruction. The surgical scrub nurse hands the surgeon a hemostat. The purpose of this instrument is to:

    a. grip tissue to provide visibility to the surgical site.
    b. control the flow of blood at the surgical site.
    c. suction blood away from the surgical field.
    d. cut away deep tissue once the surgical incision is made.

9. Which of the following does not align with the handoff process as recommended by the Joint Commission?

    a. Enhances communication and patient safety
    b. May be personalized at the preference of the reporter
    c. Signifies a transfer of provider care responsibility
    d. Is a best practice to keep team members informed

10. The nurse manager and nurse educator are reviewing the expiration dates on basic life support certificates. They realize that the certificate for one nurse shows an expiration date past due by one month. When they meet with the nurse, she exclaims, "I had no idea that the date expired! Thank you for telling me!" She promptly arranges to attend a class. The individual ultimately responsible for being aware of the expired certificate is the:

    a. nurse.
    b. nurse educator.
    c. nurse manager.
    d. BLS instructor.

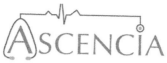

11. An 82-year-old female patient is admitted for dysphagia. She undergoes a gastrostomy tube (G tube) placement. A physician order in the electronic record states that the G tube can be used. The nurse is administering her medication and notes that the medication administration record displays the route for all of her medication as "PO," indicating the oral route. What is the next nursing action?
  a. Administer the medication orally.
  b. Administer the medication through the gastrostomy tube.
  c. Contact the physician for clarification of the medication route.
  d. Contact the pharmacy to see if the medications can be administered through the gastrostomy tube.

12. The nurse is caring for a 47-year-old male patient who experienced rib fractures as a result of a chest wall injury. As part of his treatment to manage pain, an epidural is inserted. The nurse knows that she will need to perform frequent motor and sensory assessments. Which of the following statements is most accurate about nursing management of this patient?
  a. The nurse increases the settings on the epidural pump when the block is too high because the patient is not receiving enough of the drug.
  b. The nurse performs frequent assessments of the patient's motor function because loss of motor function is a frequent complication of thoracic epidurals.
  c. Patients must be monitored closely for hypertension, which is a complication caused by constriction of smooth muscles when the patient is dehydrated.
  d. Regions of decreased sensation can be detected using a cool swab, such as an alcohol wipe, because nerves innervate skin dermatomes.

13. Which of the following is a quality outcome measure that is closely related to the discharge process?
  a. Surgical infection rate
  b. Readmission rate
  c. Number of board-certified healthcare providers
  d. Cleanliness of the facility

14. The nurse is caring for a hospice patient whose prognosis is poor. The patient has become restless and agitated. What intervention would be best for this patient's comfort?
  a. Providing range of motion
  b. Increasing stimulus to help the patient reorient
  c. Encouraging the family to leave the patient alone so they can rest
  d. Assessing oxygenation levels

15. Two nursing assistants are assigned as lunch buddies, but they are arguing about which one should break for lunch first. They go to the charge nurse and ask her to decide. The charge nurse uses a laissez-faire leadership style, which is exemplified by which statement?
  a. "What concerns do you have about the time you go to lunch?"
  b. "You go to lunch now and you go to lunch later."
  c. "Let's consider your tasks to determine the best time for you to take a break."
  d. "I'm not deciding that. You need to figure out your breaks for yourselves."

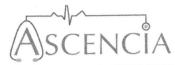

16. When delivering messages over multiple mediums, what is the most effective way to ensure that the message will be received as intended?
   a. Use slang words to connect to younger staff members
   b. Consider audience first when preparing communication style, education level, and form of medium
   c. Use a sixth to eighth grade reading level for any audience
   d. Text with emojis and abbreviations

17. A 56-year-old female patient is admitted to the nursing unit with a history of chronic back pain. The patient states that she does not want to take narcotics. The nurse aims to personalize the patient's care and implement complementary and alternative medicine (CAM) measures, which include all of the following EXCEPT:
   a. A sleep mask
   b. A consult for a nurse who specializes in reiki
   c. An analgesic adjuvant
   d. Lavender-scented spray on her pillow

18. The charge nurse is performing a daily check on the crash cart per the institutional policy. He knows that the items must be ready for a life-threatening emergency. Which of the following would raise concern regarding patient safety?
   a. The emergency equipment was checked yesterday.
   b. The oxygen tank is 1500 psi ($\frac{3}{4}$ full).
   c. The defibrillator equipment works when it is unplugged.
   d. The cart is unlocked and easily accessible.

19. Nurse leaders often practice according to a leadership philosophy, which sets the tone for the work environment. Nurse leaders who live by their philosophy and embody these principles through their words and actions are considered authentic leaders. Which action of the nurse manager is most related to authentic leadership?
   a. Performing cost-benefit analysis when considering a new product
   b. Managing conflicts among nursing staff
   c. Planning staff meetings and offering transparency when questions arise
   d. Supporting competence of nurses by ensuring certificates are up-to-date

20. A 68-year-old male patient is admitted to the medical-surgical unit with a diagnosis of cholelithiasis. He has a past medical history of chronic kidney disease, diabetes mellitus, and chronic obstructive pulmonary disease (COPD). The patient reports intermittent sharp right upper quadrant pain with diaphoresis, nausea, and vomiting. He is transferred to the operating room to undergo a cholecystectomy and will be under general anesthesia. Which of the following statements is not true about general anesthesia?
   a. Vasodilation impedes tissue oxygenation, which puts the patient at risk for a surgical site infection.
   b. Hypoxemia may be a consequence because the patient's respiratory drive is affected.
   c. Atrial fibrillation is a common risk, which may alter the patient's hemodynamic stability.
   d. Delirium may be an adverse effect because of delayed clearance of the anesthetic.

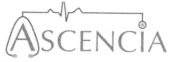

21. What is the primary focus of Quality Assurance (QA) programs in healthcare?
    a.   Elevating patient and clinical satisfaction through evidence-based interventions
    b.   Identifying areas of concern and deviations from established standards
    c.   Conducting root cause analyses to investigate occurrences
    d.   Recognizing patterns and trends in care delivery

22. The nurse is admitting a 57-year-old female patient from the post-anesthesia care unit (PACU) after she underwent a colostomy placement. He examines the colostomy and notes that the site is raised from the skin, red in color, and without stool production. When the nurse asks the patient if she has seen the site, she averts her eyes and flatly says, "No." What is the next step in the nursing process that the nurse should take?
    a.   Obtaining a mirror so that the patient has an easier time seeing the new colostomy
    b.   Providing education by printing several handouts on how to care for her colostomy at home
    c.   Documenting in the nursing notes that the patient has altered body image related to her new colostomy
    d.   Coordinating an inpatient consult with a wound, ostomy, and continence (WOC) nurse

23. The executive leadership of an organization is reviewing data regarding readmission rates. They can identify which of the following as a modifiable factor?
    a.   Prior hospitalization within the last 6 to 12 months
    b.   Bedside rounding compliance
    c.   Cancer diagnosis
    d.   Polypharmacy

24. The nurse is caring for a 15-year-old girl who came into the hospital reporting that she is hungry. She is alone and her clothes are worn and tattered. The nurse asks about her living conditions. The patient states that she lives with her mother who is depressed and stays in bed for most of the day. The nurse suspects which type of abuse?
    a.   Emotional abuse
    b.   Physical abuse
    c.   Sexual abuse
    d.   Neglect

25. A nurse has been extremely busy throughout the shift. One of her patients asks for pain medication. The nurse retrieves the tablet from the automated medication dispensing cabinet and administers the medication without scanning it. A few minutes later, the nurse notices that the patient's lips are swollen. The nurse realized the medication was stocked incorrectly in the cabinet and she had given the wrong one. The nurse manager decides to request a nursing peer review process. She explains the process to the nurse as:
    a.   a way for peers to determine the penalty required for administering the wrong medication.
    b.   a method for peers to critique all areas of the nurse's practice.
    c.   a way to support peers by identifying areas needing improvement for practice change.
    d.   a method for peers and nursing leaders to review the compliance issues with policy.

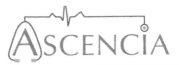

26. An 86-year-old male patient is admitted to the nursing unit. The nurse performs a neurological assessment and determines that the patient is oriented to self only. He appears to be grimacing, but he cannot communicate any details about pain. The nurse decides that the most ideal pain rating scale she should use is the:
    a. Behavioral Pain Scale.
    b. Face, Legs, Activity, Cry, Consolability (FLACC) scale.
    c. Pain Assessment in Advanced Dementia (PAINAD) scale.
    d. Wong-Baker Faces scale.

27. In which of the following circumstances would an autopsy likely be performed?
    a. 82-year-old died of natural causes
    b. 34-year-old cardiac arrest, negative for drug screen
    c. 54-year-old suicide victim
    d. 42-year-old with cancer admitted to hospice center

28. A patient is being seen in the emergency department for a cough and chest pain. What is the first step of the process through this continuum of care?
    a. Direct admission to a medical-surgical unit
    b. Triage to determine the severity of illness
    c. Treatment of the cough to see if the chest pain is relieved
    d. Sending the patient to a walk-in clinic, as a cough is not an emergency

29. Two nurses are arguing with the charge nurse at the beginning of the shift. One nurse wants a certain patient in her assignment for whom she cared yesterday. The other nurse argues that he cared for the patient several days in a row, but was off work yesterday. Which of the following does NOT characterize a collaborative style of conflict management?
    a. The nurses work together toward a solution that leads to the best outcome.
    b. Both nurses have an equal opportunity to share their point of view.
    c. Each nurse must forgo a part of their request to arrive at a solution.
    d. The solution determined is the best-case scenario that can be reached for everyone involved.

30. A nurse has paged the attending provider twice to clarify a medication order. The order is written as twice the strength as what is stated on the home medication list. The nurse waited for thirty minutes with no response. What would be the next most appropriate action for the nurse to take?
    a. Administer the medication as it is written
    b. Complain to a fellow nurse
    c. Text another provider that is a personal friend
    d. Escalate concern to the charge nurse

31. The interdisciplinary team is considering placing a central line and ordering TPN. Which of the following conditions would be the most appropriate for TPN consideration?
    a. Structural dysphagia
    b. Multiple sclerosis
    c. Prolonged ileus
    d. Patient recovering from stroke and can intake small amounts of pureed food

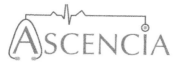

32. The preceptor notices that his new orientee is struggling to accomplish her nursing care. The new nurse reports that she is overwhelmed, but afraid to delegate any tasks to the nursing assistant because she is fully responsible for the patient. What explanation does the preceptor use to indicate that delegation is an important nursing responsibility?
   a. The nursing assistant is fully accountable for the care that is completed.
   b. The nursing assistant presumes the interventions needed for patient care.
   c. The nurse can gain time by assigning specific tasks to a nursing assistant.
   d. The nurse can best work independently by delegating to the right person.

33. Why is it crucial for researchers to properly cite all sources of information, including previously published studies, throughout the clinical research process?
   a. Citing sources is an administrative requirement but does not impact the research's integrity.
   b. Citing sources allows researchers to claim credit for others' work and ideas.
   c. Citing sources ensures transparency and provides a reference for readers to access the cited information.
   d. Citing sources is only necessary for qualitative research but not quantitative studies.

34. The nurse is caring for a 52-year-old female patient who was transferred from the intensive care unit (ICU) to the medical-surgical unit. The nurse discovers that the patient has a central venous catheter (CVC) in the right femoral vein, inserted urgently 3 days ago. Upon assessing the femoral CVC site, what is the priority action for the nurse?
   a. Gathering supplies, including sterile gloves, to change the dressing
   b. Flushing each lumen of the line to establish patency with a 10 mL syringe of 0.9% normal saline
   c. Reviewing the medical record to determine the exact date when the CVC was inserted
   d. Discussing the necessity and removal of the line with the interdisciplinary team

35. The nurse is assigned to four patients with the following characteristics. Which of the patients is most at risk for poor health literacy?
   a. 45-year-old Caucasian female
   b. 25-year-old Hispanic male who is not fluent in English
   c. 32-year-old female with three children who is currently taking college courses
   d. 68-year-old male who recently retired as an attorney

36. A nurse leader meets with his nursing staff and discusses overspending on the financial budget for the nursing unit. He would like the staff to use productive hours judiciously. This includes:
   a. not accruing incidental overtime.
   b. being mindful of the amount of office supplies used.
   c. only attending necessary education.
   d. decreasing the amount of paid time off taken.

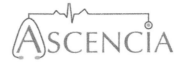

37. A 68-year-old male patient is diagnosed with pneumonia with a sputum culture positive for Methicillin-resistant *Staphylococcus aureus* (MRSA). He has a low-grade fever of 100.5 °F/38.1 °C, heart rate of 104 bpm, respiratory rate of 23 breaths per minute, blood pressure of $\frac{138}{65}$, and SaO2 of 95 percent on 2 L via nasal cannula. His lung sounds are coarse and his cough is productive with yellow sputum. The nurse is preparing an albuterol nebulizer treatment. Which personal protective equipment (PPE) should she don?

    a. Gloves, gown, mask, and face shield
    b. Gown and gloves
    c. Mask and face shield
    d. Gloves, gown, N95 mask, and face shield

38. The charge nurse overhears two nurses discussing the concept of the professional nursing role. They state that the professional nursing role is directed by the standards of care. He clarifies that the standards of care refer to:

    a. the behaviors of practice and level of competence to which all nurses adhere.
    b. the duty and responsibility that the nurse makes to her nurse manager.
    c. the policies and procedures that are outlined by the nurse's place of employment.
    d. the expectation that nurses will practice to the highest level of their ability.

39. The nurse has brought in the morning medications for a patient who has identified themselves as being Mormon. The patient is asked what they would like to drink. The nurse knows that the patient avoids what type of beverage?

    a. Non-organic
    b. Carbonated
    c. Plain water
    d. Caffeinated

40. What is the primary distinction between evidence-based practice (EBP) and clinical research in healthcare?

    a. EBP focuses on patient values and preferences, while clinical research primarily emphasizes clinical expertise.
    b. EBP involves experiments and clinical trials, while clinical research integrates current research and clinical guidelines.
    c. EBP and clinical research are interchangeable terms with no substantive differences.
    d. EBP aims to provide the most effective and safe care to patients, while clinical research generates new knowledge or validates existing evidence.

41. A new nurse is caring for a 67-year-old diabetic patient. According to his blood glucose test, the patient requires coverage per a sliding scale of regular insulin. The nurse withdraws 100 units of regular insulin and administers the amount to the patient. Afterwards, she realizes that the patient only required 10 units of insulin and she misinterpreted the vial insulin concentration for the dose. To review the events leading to the error, her manager asks her to attend which session?

    a. Root Cause Analysis
    b. Failure Mode and Effects Analysis
    c. Emergency Preparedness
    d. Value Analysis

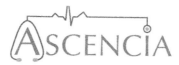

42. A patient is nearing death, and the family is asking the nurse about organ donation. The family has stated that the patient has signed to have their organs donated. What would be the most appropriate next step for the nurse?
   a. Discuss options with the family regarding organ donation
   b. Call the appropriate Organ Procure Organization per state guidelines
   c. Notify the family that the patient is not eligible to donate since they have hepatitis C
   d. Assure the family that since the patient has signed the card, all viable organs will be donated

43. A 78-year-old female patient is admitted to the hospital to undergo an elective right total knee replacement. The registered nurse (RN) circulator spends time preoperatively asking the patient about her goals with the surgery and preferences about her care. The nurse knows that understanding the patient's desires is most important because the RN circulator:
   a. works to restore the patient's health from her baseline condition.
   b. provides a handoff report to the nurse in the post-anesthesia care unit (PACU).
   c. advocates for the patient when the patient is under general anesthesia.
   d. implements the nursing interventions required and evaluates the outcomes.

44. When conducting the initial comprehensive assessment on a patient, the nurse knows the best source of information is which of the following?
   a. Patient
   b. Medical record
   c. Caregiver
   d. Family or friend

45. The healthcare executive leaders decide to open a brand-new orthopedic nursing unit and assign a director of nursing. The director is considering which nursing care delivery model to use. She believes that patient turnover will be quick, so she prefers a model that allows nurses to work with an assigned group of patients that varies by shift. She decides that the most appropriate nursing care delivery model is:
   a. functional nursing.
   b. primary care nursing.
   c. team nursing.
   d. total patient care.

46. Which of the following is an effect of poor interoperability between electronic health records?
   a. Reliance on slower methods of transmission
   b. Increased access to health records
   c. Comprehensive patient care
   d. Improved communication between different health systems

47. The nurse is about to provide teaching about the care plan to a patient with moderate hearing loss who has hearing aids but does not like to wear them. The nurse wants to ensure that the patient can hear as education is provided. What should the nurse do to enhance learning?
   a. Insist that the patient wear the hearing aids before providing education
   b. Speak in a louder tone of voice
   c. Sit closely to the patient
   d. Use visual aids such as a storyboard

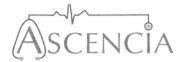

48. How can healthcare organizations best accommodate patients with blindness or significant vision loss?
   a. Ensure there is extra staff available to lead the patient around
   b. Avoid using braille on signs since the patient cannot locate them
   c. Ask the patient to bring a sign language interpreter to their appointment
   d. Incorporate large print and audio formats for educational materials

49. A nurse manager is describing the organizational disaster response to the nursing staff. What designated centralized location is the focal point for all communication that occurs during the disaster?
   a. Safety and security office
   b. Public information headquarters
   c. Logistics and resource hub
   d. Hospital command center

50. Within a Nursing Professional Practice Model, what are the core values that serve as the ethical foundation for nursing practice, and how do they impact interactions with patients and colleagues?
   a. The core values are primarily focused on administrative principles, improving management efficiency.
   b. The core values include efficiency and timeliness, ensuring a streamlined care delivery process.
   c. The core values include compassion and advocacy, promoting ethical nursing practice.
   d. The core values emphasize cost-effectiveness and resource allocation for healthcare organizations.

51. The nurse is caring for a patient who has transitioned to hospice. How can the nurse best support the patient's family in coping with the anticipated death of the patient?
   a. Adhere to strict visiting hours
   b. Tell the family that the grief will improve after the patient passes away
   c. Provide the family with a card for a local support group
   d. Arrange for a chaplain visitation, with family permission

52. When the care provider of a patient changes, what process must occur prior to the transfer of care?
   a. Punching into the timekeeping system at the start of the shift
   b. Revising the care plan prior to the new caregiver assuming care of the patient
   c. Meeting with the interdisciplinary team to review the patient's status
   d. A handoff report that includes important details on the patient's care

53. The nurse educator meets with a pharmacist and dietician to review upcoming changes regarding nasogastric tube procedures. The nurse educator knows that the devices are infrequently used and believes the nursing staff may benefit from a thorough review. She decides to conduct a learning needs assessment, which is:
   a. a way to measure an existing gap between the current practice and anticipated practice.
   b. a method used to determine how many nurses are compliant with the current policies.
   c. a plan that describes the best way to introduce a practice change so that the nurses understand.
   d. a step-by-step process by which the nurses learn the new practice changes in sequence.

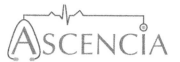

54. The nurse is caring for a 76-year-old male, transferred to the medical-surgical unit after undergoing a left hip replacement. Upon transfer, the patient is awake and alert. The nurse performs a neurological assessment, and he is oriented to person, place, time, and purpose. On postoperative day (POD) 1, the nurse finds the patient agitated. What is the priority action for the nurse?
    a. Review the medical record to determine if the patient was confused during the last shift.
    b. Use the Confusion Assessment Method (CAM) to assess whether the patient has disorganized thinking.
    c. Make sure the bed alarm is activated before leaving the room.
    d. Notify the physician that the patient is agitated and ask for a benzodiazepine order.

55. A nurse has worked the night shift on his nursing unit for approximately two years. The nurse manager asks him to take a charge nurse class because he has grown in his practice. He attends the class and learns that the charge nurse has many duties, except:
    a. being aware of the competence of each team member.
    b. giving pain medication to a patient without being asked.
    c. speaking with a daughter who has concerns about her dad's care.
    d. delegating a bed bath to a nursing assistant.

56. Which of the following is the quality outcome measure that describes an organization's systems and processes and ability to provide high-quality care?
    a. Process measures
    b. Outcome measures
    c. Optimal measures
    d. Structural measures

57. The nurse is providing education to a patient on the 2020–2025 dietary guidelines. Which of the following is promoted by the CDC as a healthy food choice?
    a. Full-fat milk
    b. Vegetables and fruits that are in the same color range
    c. Avoidance of meats
    d. Vegetarian proteins including soybeans and legumes

58. The medical-surgical nurse is admitting a patient for hyperglycemia. The patient has limited understanding and use of English and is fluent in Tagalog. A seventeen-year-old niece has accompanied her aunt and volunteers to translate. How would the nurse best support patient communication?
    a. Offer translation services
    b. Allow the niece to translate
    c. Call the charge nurse to see if there is anyone who knows Tagalog
    d. Try to continue communicating in English since the patient is nodding in response to questions

59. A 79-year-old patient is hospitalized with diverticulitis in the medical-surgical nursing unit. She is alert and oriented. She reports tenderness to the left lower quadrant and feels weak with general malaise. The nurse is concerned that her weakness may lead to falling. How can the nurse best prevent a fall with this patient?
    a. Assist the patient with ambulation in the hallway.
    b. Make sure that the patient is close to the nurse's station.
    c. Explain that the bed alarm will be enacted so that she does not get up without assistance.
    d. Delegate to the nursing assistant to perform frequent checks.

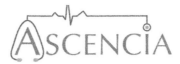

60. The nurse is caring for a patient admitted to the med-surg unit after a syncopal episode that occurred after vomiting and diarrhea. Which of the following symptoms would indicate that the patient has severe dehydration?
    a. Dry mouth
    b. Headache
    c. Fatigue
    d. Seizure

61. Which method would best show that the nurse is using active listening techniques?
    a. Asking yes and no questions to clarify patient understanding
    b. Holding conference in a public space, so the patient feels more comfortable
    c. Summarizing what the patient states and reflecting on the patient's feelings
    d. Texting patient responses to the provider to enhance interdisciplinary communication

62. Which of the following best describes upholding the patient-centered care model through the continuum of care during a hospitalization?
    a. Developing a relationship built on honest communication and trust
    b. Considering resources and socioeconomic status only for vulnerable populations
    c. Focusing on the patient's needs and preferences only within the inpatient setting
    d. Providing resources to the patient after discharge if they call to report an issue

63. On postoperative day (POD) 2, the medical-surgical nurse is caring for a patient admitted for lysis of adhesions. The nurse is concerned that the patient has a postoperative ileus, especially because the patient is experiencing which distinct sign?
    a. Abdominal distention
    b. Lack of stool
    c. Nausea and vomiting
    d. Lack of intestinal motility

64. A nurse manager meets with his nursing staff and shares that he is concerned about the turnover on the nursing unit. He asks for staff input because he wants to create a plan that can help with nurse retention. He explains that the primary concern he has related to the impact of high turnover is:
    a. the cost of training a newly licensed nurse who leaves shortly after orientation.
    b. the increasing number of patients falling with injury, according to unit quality indicators.
    c. decreasing patient satisfaction, according to patient surveys.
    d. the nurses' decreased enthusiasm for the job and how that may impact patients.

65. A med-surg nursing unit is preparing for a scheduled downtime. Which of the following would best prepare for alternate documentation?
    a. Management directive to abstain from documenting during the downtime hours
    b. Ensuring that paper charting forms are available and accessible
    c. Communicating expectations for nurses to make their own notes and then enter them after downtime is complete
    d. Delay downtime until all patients may be moved to another unit

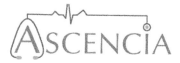

66. Beyond immediate patient harm, how can adverse events like medication errors or nosocomial infections impact healthcare facilities, and why is reporting these incidents essential to mitigate such effects?
    a. Adverse events have minimal impact on healthcare facilities, and reporting is primarily a legal requirement.
    b. Adverse events can lead to increased costs, damage to the facility's reputation, and compromised patient safety. Reporting is vital to prompt mitigation.
    c. Adverse events primarily result in staff retraining, and reporting serves as a routine administrative process.
    d. Adverse events solely affect the immediate patient and have no broader impact on healthcare facilities.

67. Which of the following is NOT a component of the SBAR communication tool?
    a. Background
    b. Status
    c. Recommendation
    d. Assessment

68. Which of the following is a barrier to a healthcare organization improving bicultural representation of their community?
    a. Incentives to attract a diverse pool of healthcare staff
    b. A high migrant population in the community
    c. Policy that mandates culturally competent education for staff
    d. C-Suite leadership hiring based solely on years of experience

69. The RN is precepting a new grad RN and asks her to observe the vascular access nurse insert a peripherally inserted central catheter (PICC) line. The RN explains that the preceptee must perform hand hygiene prior to inserting the line, then adhere to aseptic technique to prevent infection. What else does he include in his teaching that can reduce the risk of a central line-associated bloodstream infection (CLABSI)?
    a. A mask and clean gown must first be obtained from the supply closet for donning.
    b. The door to the patient room should be closed during the procedure.
    c. The insertion site should be prepared with betadine.
    d. All of the above is appropriate for standard CLABSI prevention standards.

70. The medical-surgical nurse is caring for an 82-year-old postoperative male patient who underwent an open cholecystectomy after an attempt at laparoscopic surgery was not successful. The patient is oriented at baseline but is currently pleasantly confused. Which of the following interventions should the nurse NOT implement?
    a. Promoting sleep by administering temazepam (Restoril) short-term
    b. Creating an ambulation schedule of at least three times in the hallway
    c. Asking the daughter to visit the patient as much as possible
    d. Exposing the patient to natural lighting during the day

71. When is the ideal time frame for education to begin on new treatment with the patient and family?
    a. After the treatment has begun
    b. During the discharge process
    c. When the treatment is initially proposed by the care team
    d. Once the patient is within their home environment

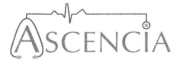

72. A new nurse manager is attending a leadership seminar about conflict management. She learns that since conflicts often arise in the workplace, conflict management is an important strength. In fact, managing conflict on the nursing unit is MOST important because:
    a. the nursing team must work together to deliver effective quality of care to the patient.
    b. although conflict is unavoidable, sometimes positive changes may result.
    c. when there is better morale among the nursing staff, it creates a positive working environment.
    d. there is less staff turnover among the nursing staff, and nurses are more satisfied with their jobs.

73. Which aspect of the "5 C's" framework emphasizes the importance of maintaining ongoing, consistent relationships between patients and their healthcare providers?
    a. Continuity
    b. Consistency
    c. Coordination
    d. Caring

74. The nurse is caring for a 73-year-old male patient admitted to the hospital for intractable back pain that has slowly improved since his admission. The patient requests pain medication after he rates the pain as $\frac{5}{10}$ on the Numerical Pain Scale. The nurse administers prescribed ibuprofen. Upon reassessment, the patient reports no relief. According to the analgesic ladder, what pain intervention should the nurse use next?
    a. Acetaminophen
    b. Codeine
    c. Hydromorphone
    d. A heating pad

75. The nurse has been taking care of a patient with a fractured leg that has progressed from traction. The interdisciplinary team has discussed discharge occurring within the next week. The patient's spouse expresses concern that she does not have the strength or support to take care of him at home. What is the nurse's best course of action to facilitate discharging the patient?
    a. Assure the spouse that she will find ways to take care of the patient at home
    b. Request an order for intermittent home care three times per week
    c. Contact the social worker for guidance on rehabilitation facility placement
    d. Encourage the patient to do as much as possible to relieve the burden on the spouse

76. A 56-year-old patient underwent a total hip replacement. His postoperative assessment shows a large clean, dry, and intact dressing to his left hip. The nurse reviews the postoperative orders. What nursing intervention would aid in the prevention of a surgical site infection?
    a. Removing the dressing to further assess the incision site for any redness, inflammation, or exudate
    b. Providing the patient with a warm blanket when the patient complains of feeling cold
    c. Continuously monitoring the patient's integumentary status
    d. Encouraging the use of an incentive spirometer

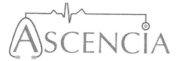

77. What age category is the Wong-Baker FACES Pain Rating Scale aimed to be used for?
   a. Infant
   b. Toddler
   c. Adolescents
   d. All age ranges

78. The medical-surgical nurse is caring for a patient who has developed erythema and a heart rate of 95 beats per minute after a scheduled dose of IV vancomycin. The nurse has stopped the infusion. What is the next best step if the nurse remains concerned regarding the potential reaction?
   a. Call a code blue
   b. Contact the charge nurse to initiate a rapid response
   c. Leave the patient to retrieve an EpiPen
   d. Wait a few minutes to see if the patient improves

79. A nurse is caring for a newly diagnosed diabetic patient. When he initiates patient education, he uses the teach-back technique. The nurse feels that this is most appropriate for the patient because:
   a. the patient can explain the content back to the nurse using her own words.
   b. the nurse can quiz the patient's knowledge to see how well she remembers the information.
   c. the patient can easily use yes or no responses instead of giving longer answers.
   d. teach-back takes time to implement, and the nurse can thoroughly review the education.

80. The healthcare facility's emergency response has been activated. The hospital is expecting to receive a large number of victims due to an earthquake. While triaging, a patient presents with a closed arm fracture that he sustained when the wall of the building collapsed in his workplace. According to the triage classification system, the nurse knows that this patient is classified as:
   a. wounded.
   b. non-urgent.
   c. urgent.
   d. emergent.

81. Which phase of the project development model involves the practical implementation of the project plan, including tasks such as introducing new clinical protocols or healthcare technology systems in a healthcare context?
   a. Initiation
   b. Planning
   c. Execution
   d. Monitoring/controlling

82. The nurse is caring for a patient with congestive heart failure who develops hemoptysis, shortness of breath, and hypoxemia. The nurse calls the healthcare provider and prepares to use SBAR to communicate the concerns. What component should be a part of the Assessment?
   a. Medical history
   b. Urgency of event
   c. Nursing judgment of reason for event
   d. Action that needs to occur to improve clinical status

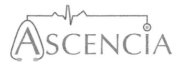

83. How can incorporating spirituality into hospice care affect patient outcomes?
    a. Increases guilt, thereby increasing compliance
    b. Assists patient with decision making
    c. Increases anxiety regarding death
    d. Increases depressive symptoms

84. An 87-year-old male patient undergoes a surgical wound debridement after experiencing a nonhealing surgical incision following a right total hip replacement 6 weeks ago. The medical-surgical nurse reviews an order for the vascular access team to insert a peripherally inserted central venous catheter (PICC) line so that the patient can receive long-term antibiotics and have lab draws. Which of the following does the medical-surgical nurse NOT anticipate?
    a. The medical-surgical nurse will perform a timeout with the vascular access nurse at the bedside prior to insertion.
    b. The tip of the PICC line will be confirmed by an electrocardiogram-guided PICC placement.
    c. The patient will require a limb restriction wristband to alert other staff members about the line.
    d. The patient is at high risk for a pneumothorax, the most common complication of a PICC line.

85. The nurse leader is evaluating the work environment in the med-surg nursing unit. She is concerned about the staff morale and feels that she can improve teamwork and other components of a healthy work environment. What is one measure that she would NOT include?
    a. There must be sufficiently stocked personal protective equipment (PPE).
    b. Staff should be assigned mandatory overtime when a nurse calls out sick to ensure adequate compensation.
    c. There must be puncture-free sharps containers available to protect from injury.
    d. Staff should be trained to move patients in a safe manner.

86. A wound committee is planning a quality initiative project with the support of nurse executive leaders. They are introducing a new mattress to reduce hospital-acquired pressure injuries. One of the nurse leaders believes the mattress should be piloted on one of the units before being distributed to all units. She wants to know how the change will affect the workflow. In which step of the ADKAR change theory will piloting the mattress be planned?
    a. Awareness
    b. Desire
    c. Knowledge
    d. Ability

87. Which of the following is the best approach for providing pain relief in palliative and hospice care?
    a. Strong opioids
    b. Multi-modal
    c. Pharmacological only
    d. Solely non-opioid to prevent addiction

88. Which of the following is a barrier to patient hand-offs?
    a. Time limitations
    b. Standardization of reporting
    c. Patient family participation
    d. Adhering to HIPAA standards

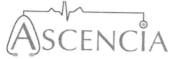

89. When planning an educational session for a patient, what should the nurse first consider?
    a. The patient's preferred style of learning
    b. Whether the patient has college education
    c. The time that is available for the educational session
    d. Whether the patient already has the knowledge of the education that is going to be provided

90. Which of the following is NOT a characteristic of subconscious bias?
    a. Always negative assumptions
    b. May not be based on reality
    c. Unconscious
    d. Can predict behaviors

91. The nurse is responding to a malignant hyperthermia drill announced in the intensive care unit. On arrival to the room, the scenario is described as the patient's temperature increasing rapidly after undergoing a total abdominal hysterectomy. Her vital signs show a temperature of 104°F, heart rate of 145, respiratory rate of 26, and blood pressure of $\frac{185}{100}$. Upon debriefing about the drill, the nurse is questioned about the pathophysiology of malignant hyperthermia. She states that the mechanism for malignant hyperthermia is:
    a. a massive release of calcium by the skeletal muscle cells.
    b. a magnesium insufficiency that leads to a hypoactive muscular state.
    c. cancer cells that cause deregulation of the hypothalamus.
    d. a metabolic state of hyperkalemia producing tall peaked T waves.

92. When a patient is being discharged with a referral for post-hospitalization services, which of the following information should the nurse provide the patient with?
    a. A list of agencies based on the nurse's opinion
    b. The cost of treatment based on the patient's insurance
    c. The referral agency will provide the patient with all information needed.
    d. The name and contact information for the agency, if known

93. In order for an advance directive to be considered legally binding, what action must be completed?
    a. Signed by an attorney
    b. Filed with the courthouse
    c. Notarized
    d. Signed by the proxy

94. The nurse is admitting an elderly woman who appears very frail and fatigued. The doctor requests that she undergoes numerous tests to determine the cause, but she seems reluctant. The nurse sits down beside her and asks, "Would you prefer that we help make you comfortable?" She adamantly agrees. A few hours later, she passes away. The nurse keeps recalling in his mind the details of the event, how he felt, and if he should have done something differently. This activity is called:
    a. clinical reasoning.
    b. professional engagement.
    c. professional empowerment.
    d. reflective practice.

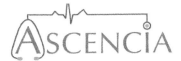

95. What is a technique that can decrease errors in delivering and receiving a verbal provider order?
  a. Closed-loop communication
  b. Active listening
  c. Summarizing
  d. Reflecting

96. What tool can be used to identify gaps in care to improve cultural and linguistic needs?
  a. Risk assessment
  b. Patient survey
  c. Staff interviews
  d. Provider opinions

97. The nurse is finishing her shift and is preparing to give the handoff report to the oncoming nurse. The charge nurse calls a safety huddle and encourages all available staff to attend. The nurse knows that the purpose of the huddle is to accomplish which of the following?
  a. Communicating safety issues and solving problems together
  b. Discussing safety issues with upper management
  c. Sharing safety concerns in anticipation of the upcoming shift
  d. Thoroughly reviewing safety concerns from last week

98. The nurse is caring for a 42-year-old female who underwent a Roux-en-Y gastric bypass surgery. On postoperative day 2, the nurse assesses the patient's vital signs. The results include a temperature of 100.9°F/38.2°C and respiratory rate of 20. The patient has decreased breath sounds and white sputum production. What action should the nurse perform first?
  a. Administer acetaminophen so that the patient's temperature decreases.
  b. Assist the patient out of bed and encourage her to ambulate in the hallway.
  c. Gather supplies to take a wound culture from the incision site.
  d. Monitor the patient's vital signs by reassessing her in 2 hours.

99. The nurse is caring for a patient recovering from a gastrostomy insertion who is being transferred back to the adult care facility that they reside at. The nurse has notified and given a standardized report to the emergency medical services team for transport. What other informational tactic should be used to facilitate safe patient care?
  a. Standardized report form
  b. Report to family to relay to adult care facility staff
  c. Full copy of the patient's medical record
  d. Medication reconciliation list

100. The nurse works at a healthcare facility that uses a hierarchical structure with the chief nurse officer (CNO) acting as the executive leader. The nurse understands that the CNO prioritizes her responsibilities by:
  a. advising how orientation can be structured to meet planned organizational goals.
  b. determining the financial and scheduling needs for the nursing unit to retain staff.
  c. creating all the policies and procedures for the nursing department.
  d. overseeing the new technology and supplies for the medical-surgical units.

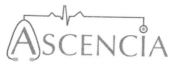

101. Which of the following interdisciplinary communications is considered formal?
    a. Memo
    b. Note on chart
    c. Casual face-to-face conversation
    d. Facility-wide forum presented by leadership

102. Which of the following is a common barrier in communication with the patient-provider relationship?
    a. Socioeconomic status
    b. Disadvantaged groups
    c. Differing native language
    d. Large age gap

103. The nursing unit decides to take on a project to decrease catheter-associated urinary tract infections (CAUTI). The nurse leaders review current literature, calculate the CAUTI rate, and purchase standardized urinary catheters. Queries are added to the nursing documentation prompting the nurses to inquire about the catheter necessity and keep track of the insertion date. A large nursing education initiative was also planned. These actions best represent:
    a. evidence-based practice.
    b. Root Cause Analysis.
    c. Failure Mode and Effect Analysis.
    d. lean healthcare.

104. The medical-surgical nurse is caring for a 32-year-old female patient who underwent a total abdominal hysterectomy 3 days ago. The nurse receives orders to discontinue the indwelling urinary catheter because the epidural was discontinued when the anesthesiologist rounded. The nurse responds to the patient's call light about 6 hours after the catheter was removed, and the patient requests a bedpan. What is the nurse's best response?
    a. "That is good you need to urinate so soon. I will get that for you!"
    b. "I am going to bring the bladder scanner to check the post-void residual."
    c. "I will assist you out of bed and help you walk to the toilet."
    d. "You may not have to urinate this soon since an epidural often causes urinary retention."

105. Which of the following is a consequence to the organization of high readmission rates?
    a. High patient satisfaction
    b. Improved patient outcomes
    c. Financial penalties
    d. Trust of the community

106. A nurse manager is concerned about the number of falls with injuries that have occurred recently on her medical-surgical unit. She knows that an organizational goal is to improve patient fall rates. She is interested in decreasing falls through a mobility program. In order to share her ideas, she meets with the nursing staff and asks for volunteers to be part of a committee that investigates the possibilities. The nurse manager is using a leadership style known as:
    a. democratic.
    b. servant.
    c. transactional.
    d. transformational.

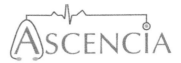

107. The nurse has participated in continuing education on inclusivity and bias. The nurse demonstrates an understanding of bias by stating which of the following?
    a. Implicit bias is always negative.
    b. Explicit bias is unconscious and unrealized.
    c. Explicit bias may include sexual harassment and work assignments or promotions due to favoritism.
    d. Bias does not affect decision-making processes.

108. The nurse manager reviews emergency preparedness with her staff. She explains the location of the Emergency Operations Plan. One nurse raises her hand and asks, "What exactly is the Emergency Operations Plan?" The nurse manager reviews its purpose in depth. Which of the following would NOT be included in this review of the Emergency Operations Plan?
    a. The structure for the response to all hazards
    b. A method of notifying staff that there is an emergency
    c. The exact steps for what will happen during the emergency
    d. The exact steps for providing effective care for patients with minimal disruption

109. A newly admitted 68-year-old male patient arrives to the nursing unit with a medical history of chronic kidney disease, congestive heart failure (CHF), chronic obstructive pulmonary disease (COPD), and depression. The patient has an extensive medication list. The pharmacist has the primary responsibility of collecting the patient data for the medication reconciliation process. The nurse's priority role in medication reconciliation on admission for this patient is to:
    a. document the last time the patient took his medication in the patient's medical record.
    b. provide teach-back education on the clinical indication for each medication.
    c. notify the provider that the patient's multivitamin is missing from the medication list.
    d. ensure that the provider orders the most cost-effective medication with the highest benefit.

110. What is the recommended sodium intake for individuals with mild cardiac disease?
    a. <3000 mg/day
    b. 4000 mg/day
    c. <2000 mg/day
    d. 1000 mg/day

111. If a patient codes and does not have an advance directive, which of the following would be consulted for ongoing medical care?
    a. Patient's personal lawyer
    b. Patient's physician
    c. Divorced spouse
    d. Sibling

112. The nursing staff is asked to enroll in an active shooter drill as part of the emergency response plan. During the education, the nurses are informed that these scenarios are important because active shooters often act impulsively and unpredictably. The drill introduces strategies for how the nurses can best protect themselves. This phase of disaster planning is called:
    a. awareness.
    b. preparedness.
    c. response.
    d. recovery.

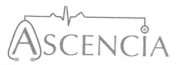

113 An 82-year-old female is admitted with a history of dementia. The admission nurse observes that the patient is getting increasingly anxious and voices that she wants to go home. The nurse completes her admission assessment, puts the bed alarm on, and leaves the room. A few minutes later, the nurse responds to the alarm sounding and finds the patient standing next to the bed trying to get dressed with the intention of going home. Which measure can the nurse best implement to prevent the patient from eloping?
   a. Urgent application of soft wrist restraints to the patient
   b. Obtaining an order to administer medication to relieve the patient's anxiety
   c. Taking the patient for a walk
   d. Assisting the patient back into bed and placing the bed alarm on

114. A 63-year-old male patient is admitted for pneumonia. He has a history of multiple myeloma and has an implanted port for chemotherapy. The nurse obtains an order that the port may be accessed for antibiotic administration and lab draws. Upon performing hand hygiene and donning the appropriate personal protective equipment (PPE), the nurse attaches the non-coring needle to the flushed extension set to the needleless connector and scrubs the access site with chlorhexidine. What is the nurse's next step to access the port?
   a. Palpate the port with the dominant gloved hand.
   b. Palpate the port with the nondominant gloved hand.
   c. Stabilize the port body with the dominant gloved hand.
   d. Stabilize the port body with the nondominant gloved hand.

115. A nurse is meeting with her nurse manager about opportunities for growth. She values patient care and has a lot of ideas for the nursing department. The manager suggests that she join one of the hospital-wide shared governance councils. How does she best explain shared governance to the nurse?
   a. A dedicated meeting that focuses on increasing leadership skills among staff to help with job retention
   b. A collaboration among nursing staff and leaders to make decisions within the organization
   c. A time allotted to different nursing units to discuss the sharing of patient care responsibilities
   d. A collective gathering that determines that all procedures within the organization are evidence-based

116. The nurse is caring for a patient who is hard of hearing with limited verbal communication. The nurse decides to try using a communication board to understand the patient's needs. Which of the following would improve the use of this alternative communication care to understand a wide variety of the patient's needs?
   a. Smaller pictures in order to fit more on one board
   b. Complex concepts
   c. Incorporate feelings, daily needs, and requests that are easy to understand
   d. Establish a time limit that the patient may use the board

117. A patient who had a tracheostomy tube insertion 1 week ago is hesitant to participate in care. The expectation is that the patient will be managing care once discharged. What strategy may the nurse encourage to assist with the patient's acceptance of the new medical device?
   a. Insist that the patient complete all care related to the tracheostomy tube
   b. Provide all care as the patient is requesting
   c. Allow the patient time to adjust and incrementally increase care involvement
   d. Only teach the patient's family the new routine of care

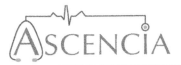

118. The medical-surgical nurse received bedside handoff upon accepting a patient transfer from the intensive care unit (ICU). The patient underwent a triple lumen central venous catheter (CVC) placement, inserted urgently after experiencing a large amount of blood loss from colonoscopy complications. When the nurse attempts to flush one of the CVC lumens, he notes an occlusion of the line. What is the nurse's priority nursing action?

    a. Administer a low-dose fibrinolytic agent by instilling the drug into the occluded port.

    b. Inspect the external catheter to see how the lumen is secured to the patient.

    c. Reposition the patient by asking him to raise his arms and turn from side to side.

    d. There is no action needed at this time because the patient has two functioning lumens.

119. When the nurse manager asks for staff input about how the nursing unit can retain nurses, the nurses share several ideas with him. All the ideas were valid, except one he believed was least related to retention, which was:

    a. avoiding the admission of patients with difficult family members.

    b. sending notes of appreciation to the nurse's home for a job well done.

    c. doing a comparative salary analysis among staff nurses within the region.

    d. providing opportunities for education on conditions with which the nurses are not familiar.

120. What healthcare maintenance practice can a nurse teach a patient that will improve cardiac function, reduce the risk of developing diabetes, and assist in weight control?

    a. Severe, restricted diet of 1400 calories per day

    b. Aerobic activity for thirty minutes a day for five days per week

    c. Weight training one time per week

    d. Consult with a dietician

121. A patient is discussing emergency care and code status with the healthcare provider. The patient states that they may want chest compressions but do not want to be intubated or defibrillated. Which of the following code statuses would be best ordered for this patient?

    a. Do not resuscitate

    b. Limited Code

    c. Full Code

    d. No status is ordered as the patient is healthy and does not need to worry

122. The nurse is working on her shift when the charge nurse announces a mock downtime drill. The nurse understands that the drill is important for which of the following reasons?

    a. The staff need to know where the emergency equipment is located.

    b. Medication errors are more prone to occur during downtime.

    c. The nurses will need to properly store any excess equipment in the hallways.

    d. The staff need to understand how to observe the stairwells for any suspicious activity.

123. The nurse manager meets with his nursing staff. He shares that he attended a nursing leadership meeting in which the strategic plan for the upcoming year was brainstormed. A nurse interjects, "What is a strategic plan?" The nurse manager best describes this concept by stating that a strategic plan is:

    a. an assessment of organizational strengths and weaknesses that identifies opportunities for growth.

    b. an inspired vision that the nurse manager role models and motivates his staff to work toward.

    c. a blueprint to support decision-making for steering the organization towards goals.

    d. a statement that describes how the organization will be providing care to the community.

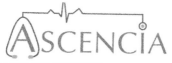

124. Which of the following statements is true regarding a medication reconciliation?
   a. Without a proper medication reconciliation process, the patient is at risk for readmission.
   b. The pharmacist completing the medication reconciliation can call the patient's pharmacy for a full list of medications if the patient forgets the names.
   c. The physician is actively involved with medication reconciliation on admission because all the patient's home medications need to be ordered in the hospital.
   d. During data collection on admission, prescribed medications are the only medications that the pharmacist needs to document.

125. An 86-year-old male admitted with exacerbation of COPD is being discharged home with oxygen by ambulance. The nurse is preparing the paperwork for the transfer. Because transitions in care can present an opportunity for a lapse in patient safety, what can the nurse best do to prepare for a successful discharge?
   a. Provide detailed instructions on the patient's new medication to the ambulance driver.
   b. Explain to the patient that he needs to make a follow up appointment with his pulmonologist.
   c. Wait until the patient is ready to leave, then review everything he needs to know.
   d. Use teach-back to assess the patient's understanding of his oxygen.

Answer Explanations #2

1. B: Reviewing existing literature and studies related to a chosen research topic is essential to build a foundation of knowledge and understand the current state of knowledge on the topic. This background information helps researchers identify gaps in knowledge, formulate hypotheses, and design their research studies effectively. Choices *A*, *C*, and *D* do not accurately represent the primary purpose of this step in the research process.

2. C: The correct answer is Choice *C*. Effective communication techniques can readily identify patient concerns through active listening and assist staff in responding empathetically. This ensures that concerns are understood and more likely to be addressed in a manner that is satisfactory to the patient. Choice *A* is not correct as a proactive stance reduces the probability of patient complaints, not a retroactive approach. Choice *B* is incorrect as patient-centered care promotes active listening. Choice *D* is not correct; the primary focus should be on providing solutions that prevent concerns from escalating, not aiming for forgiveness through reparations.

3. B: The answer is Choice *B*. Orientation is a time for developing knowledge and competence in the nurse's clinical setting to best care for patients. The other answers are not the best response. Although orientation builds upon knowledge the nurse gained in nursing school, she would not be tested on all the content she acquired there. The nurse would be accountable for her practice in orientation. Orientation supports the nurse's transition into clinical practice, but she would not learn everything she needs to know during that time.

4. D: The correct answer is Choice *D*. A surgical site infection is most related to the length of surgery lasting longer than expected. Other environmental factors are the operating room temperature, administration of cool intravenous fluids, and anesthetic drug administration. The patient's body mass index (BMI) is normal. The other options, supplemental oxygen and providing a warming blanket, are interventions implemented to anticipate temperature loss and prevent a surgical site infection.

5. D: Choice *D* is correct as the durable power of attorney is an individual designated in a legally binding document to make financial decisions on behalf of the patient if the patient is unable to make these decisions. Choice *A* is incorrect as the individual assigned to make healthcare decisions for the patient is the healthcare proxy. Choice *B* is incorrect as this is a legally binding document. Choice *C* is incorrect as the patient may choose at will who they want to represent them; however, there are some ethical considerations.

6. D: The correct answer is Choice *D*. To treat the compromised skin, the nurse may place a dressing between the ear and the device. Applying a thin layer of water-based lubricant is typically advised for patients who have soreness or irritation within the nostrils due to the prongs. Removing the oxygen solely for erythema behind the ears would not be medically appropriate, even with continuous monitoring in place. Lastly, while tightening the nasal cannula tubing can prevent skin breakdown related to friction, once there is already compromised skin, the skin should be protected with a skin barrier.

7. B: The correct answer is Choice *B* as the bedside report incorporates the patient into the hand-off by providing an overview of the plan of care, reviewing medications, and verifying vital signs and labs. The patient is introduced to the oncoming nurse and is encouraged to participate and ask questions. Choice

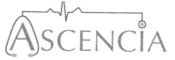

A is incorrect as it is missing the verbal component of a safe patient hand-off. Choice *C* is incorrect as it is a tool used to update and voice concerns to a healthcare provider. Choice *D* is incorrect as this is meant to update the entire healthcare team rather than provide a hand-off of pertinent information for the receiving nurse to be able to provide competent care.

8. B: The correct answer is Choice *B*. A hemostat controls bleeding by clamping or clipping a vein or artery to provide hemostasis. During surgery, hemostasis is important to stop blood flow to provide visibility to the surgical field and reduce wound complications related to bleeding.

9. B: Choice *B* is correct, as the Joint Commission advocates for a standardized report to maintain consistency of information. Choices *A*, *C*, and *D* are all in alignment with the Joint Commission's statement on reporting responsibility during transfer of care in the inpatient and outpatient setting.

10. A: The answer is Choice *A*, as the nurse is ultimately responsible for maintaining her own competencies, skillset, knowledge, nursing license, and certificates.

11. C: The correct answer is Choice *C*. The nurse should contact the physician for clarification of the medication route. The patient exhibits signs of dysphagia and therefore cannot take medication orally. When considering the five rights of medication administration, the nurse is verifying the right route.

12. D: The correct answer is Choice *D*. The nurse performs a sensory assessment using a cool swab to detect areas of decreased sensation. The other options are not the most accurate. A block that is too high indicates that there is too much of the drug. Loss of motor function is rare with a thoracic epidural and more common with a lower lumbar site. A common complication of epidurals is hypotension, caused by the effect of the epidural drug on the sympathetic nervous system.

13. B: Choice *B* is correct, as the readmission rate has been closely tied to an appropriate and timely discharge that has provided adequate education and resources for optimal outcomes post-discharge. Choice *A* may contribute to a readmission but is incorrect because it is not directly caused by the discharge process. Choices *C* and *D* are incorrect, as they are outcome measures that align with patient satisfaction, not readmission rates.

14. D: Choice *D* is correct as hypoxemia may induce terminal agitation, and oxygen treatment is appropriate for the patient's comfort. Choices *A* and *B* are not correct as overstimulating the patient may aggravate symptoms. Choice *C* is not correct as family should be encouraged to be with the patient to provide comfort and familiarity in their last hours or days.

15. D: The answer is Choice *D*. A laissez-faire leadership style is a hands-off approach. The leader avoids the situation and offers little supervision.

16. B: The correct answer is Choice *B* as communication should be tailored to the intended audience and the type of message delivered. Choice *A* is incorrect as slang may not be understood across factors such as age, culture, and language norms. Choice *C* is incorrect as meaningful communication may be delivered based on the education level of the audience. The education level will differ for education delivered to health professionals versus patients, which should be kept at a sixth to eighth grade reading level. Choice *D* is incorrect; all communication should be kept professional and abbreviations should be avoided as they can cause confusion and increase the risk of a misunderstanding.

17. C: The correct answer is Choice *C*. Complementary and alternative medicine (CAM) measures are non-pharmacological pain therapies to support pain relief. An adjuvant is a drug that may offer analgesic effects or enhance treatment when used with pain-relieving medications.

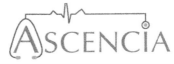

18. D: The correct answer is Choice D. Carts should be secure and inaccessible to any individual without the credentials (i.e., some units have a lock or a passcode). This prevents equipment from being touched and removed. The frequency of checking code carts is done according to organizational policy. Because the code cart was checked yesterday and the charge nurse is performing a daily check, this is within policy. Empty oxygen tanks and drained batteries are two reasons for safety-related events, along with outdated supplies, missing equipment, and incorrectly sized products.

19. C: The answer is Choice C. The nurse manager plans staff meetings and offers transparency when questions arise. Authentic leaders build trusting relationships and a healthy work environment through effective communication.

20. A: The correct answer is Choice A. Vasoconstriction, not vasodilation, impedes tissue oxygenation, which can impair wound healing and put the patient at risk for surgical site infections.

21. B: Quality Assurance (QA) programs in healthcare primarily focus on systematically monitoring and assessing care quality, with the goal of identifying areas of concern, deviations from established standards, and potential issues that require attention and improvement. Choice A is a primary goal of Performance Improvement (PI) projects, which often result from QA efforts but are distinct in their focus on implementing interventions to enhance satisfaction. Although Choice C is an important component of both QA and PI, as it helps in understanding the causes of issues and incidents, it is not the primary focus of QA programs. Choice D is another key function of QA programs because they involve recognizing patterns and trends that may indicate areas for improvement in care delivery. However, it is also not the primary focus of QA programs.

22. C: The answer is Choice C. After the nurse assesses the site and collects subjective and objective data, the nurse will make a diagnosis. In this case, the nurse determines that the patient has altered body image. The next steps would be establishing, implementing, and evaluating the plan.

23. B: Choice B is correct, as implementing bedside rounding is a best practice that can have a positive effect on improving readmission rates. Choices A, C, and D are all nonmodifiable factors.

24. D: The correct choice is Choice D. Children who are neglected do not have basic needs met, such as food, clothing, and basic safety. Emotional abuse occurs when the child is subject to yelling or humiliation. Signs of physical abuse may be bruising, bite marks, or burns. Sexual abuse may appear as injury around the genitalia or torn underwear.

25. C: The answer is Choice C. Nursing peer review is a way to support peers by identifying areas needing improvement for practice change. Considerations are skill set, stage of practice, policies, education, knowledge, and confounding factors. The process is nonpunitive. The process would not involve critiquing all areas of the nurse's practice or include nursing leaders.

26. C: The correct answer is Choice C. The Pain Assessment in Advanced Dementia (PAINAD) scale is used for patients with advanced dementia and quantifies pain through assessment of breathing character, negative vocalization, facial expression, body language, and consolability. The Behavioral Pain Scale is used for patients requiring ventilation. The Face, Legs, Activity, Cry, Consolability (FLACC) scale is typically used for patients under the age of 3. The Wong-Baker Faces scale could be tried, but the PAINAD tool is a better objective measurement.

27. C: Choice C is correct as laws mandate that patients who have suffered accidents, suicides, or homicides have an autopsy performed. Choices A, B, and D do not meet the criteria for needing an autopsy.

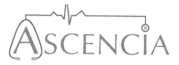

28. B: Choice *B* is correct, as all patients being treated in the emergency department will be assessed for the severity of the illness and seen in order of most to least emergent. The patient will be stabilized and reassessed to determine the plan of care. Choice *A* is not correct, as the patient needs to be assessed and diagnostic testing completed to rule out an acute diagnosis that may be life-threatening. Choice *C* is not correct, as identifying the source of the chest pain is the priority. Choice *D* is not correct, as all patients who present at the emergency department must be triaged and assessed prior to appropriate treatment and discharge planning.

29. C: The answer is Choice *C*. All the other options relate to a collaborative style of conflict management. The requirement that each nurse forgo part of their desires to arrive at a solution is part of a compromising style.

30. D: The correct answer is Choice *D* as unresolved patient concerns will require the nurse to utilize the chain of command for resolution. Choice *A* may be unsafe and cause the patient harm. Administering the dose twice when it is not intended is a medication error. Choice *B* is incorrect as it will not provide a solution to the problem. Choice *C* is incorrect because a provider that is a personal friend is not part of the patient's care team, and this would result in a HIPAA violation.

31. C: The correct answer is Choice *C*; patients who do not have gastrointestinal function that stems from disorder in the movement of nutrition through the digestive system or intestinal malabsorption are candidates for TPN. Choice *A* is incorrect as structural dysphagia involves the movement of food to and through the esophagus; this may be bypassed via NG or G-tube to deliver food to the stomach. Choice *B* is not correct as multiple sclerosis has a weakening effect on muscles and swallowing, not on the passage of food through the stomach. Choice *D* is not correct as the patient is recovering from a stroke and has some swallowing function. Supplemental enteral nutrition would be more appropriate for this patient.

32. C: The answer is Choice *C*, as delegating is an effective time management strategy. The nurse can gain time by assigning delegable tasks to the nursing assistant so she can undertake responsibilities that cannot be delegated. The other responses are not an appropriate part of delegation. Although the nursing assistant is accountable for the work delegated, the nurse is also fully accountable for the care that is completed. The nursing assistant does not presume the tasks to complete because direction is provided by the nurse. Delegation leads to better teamwork, not working independently.

33. C: Properly citing all sources of information, including previously published studies, is essential in clinical research to ensure transparency, give credit to the original authors, and provide a reference for readers to access the cited information. It upholds ethical and academic standards and allows others to verify the research's validity by reviewing the sources. Choices *A*, *B*, and *D* do not accurately represent the significance of citing sources in the research process.

34. D: The correct answer is Choice *D*. The nurse should determine the necessity of the femoral CVC line and advocate for its removal. The femoral line puts the patient at risk for infection and thrombus. The other actions are important but not the priority.

35. B: Choice *B* is the correct answer, as having a non-English native language increases risk for poor health literacy more than the other choices. Choice *A* is incorrect, as Caucasian individuals have a decreased risk. Choice *C* is incorrect, as this individual has some advanced education, which may aid in health literacy. Although being over 60 is a risk factor, Choice *D* is incorrect because this individual has a higher level of education.

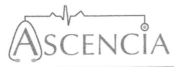

36. A: The answer is Choice *A*. Productive hours are the hours the nurse works providing direct patient care. Incidental overtime can greatly affect a budget when nurses work more than their intended shift, either arriving before or leaving after their scheduled hours. The other choices of education and paid time off are nonproductive hours, which occur when the nurse does not provide direct care. Office supplies are considered non-salary cost items.

37. A: The correct choice is Choice *A*. The PPE most appropriate for MRSA is contact precautions and face protection because the organism is identified in the sputum. The nurse should protect herself against respiratory secretions and splashes by using the appropriate precautions of gloves, gown, mask, and face shield.

38. A: The answer is Choice *A*. Standards of care are the behaviors of practice and level of competence by which all nurses adhere. The standards are set forth by the state Nurse Practice Act and adopted by professional nursing bodies.

39. D: The correct answer is Choice *D*; Mormons refrain from consuming beverages containing caffeine and alcohol. Choices *A*, *B*, and *C* are not restricted from consumption in the Mormon faith.

40. D: Evidence-based practice (EBP) focuses on providing effective and safe care to patients by integrating the best available evidence, clinical expertise, and patient values and preferences. Clinical research, on the other hand, primarily involves systematic investigation to generate new knowledge or validate existing evidence. Choices *A*, *B*, and *C* do not accurately capture the primary distinction between EBP and clinical research in healthcare.

41. A: The correct answer is Choice *A*. A Root Cause Analysis (RCA) is a quality improvement method that seeks to identify the root cause of an issue when there is harm or breakdown in care. Failure Mode and Effects Analysis (FMEA) analyzes events or problems of potential harm before it occurs. While emergency preparedness training is important, it is not relevant to this situation involving a medication error. Value Analysis would involve the review of the formulary of products (i.e., medical equipment, supplies).

42. B: Choice *B* is correct because federal law mandates that the conversation regarding organ harvesting is completed by trained professionals represented by certified Organ Procurement Organizations. Choice *A* is incorrect, as the nurse is not a trained professional in organ procurement per federal law. Choice *C* is incorrect, as even with some disease processes, corneas may be donated. Choice *D* is incorrect, as organ harvesting and viability must be assessed by the organ harvesting team.

43. C: The correct answer is Choice *C*. All of the options are responsibilities of the RN circulator, but the most relevant one for the context is Choice *C*. The RN circulator determines the patient's preferences and goals so that she can advocate for the patient when she is under general anesthesia.

44. A: Choice *A* is correct, as the patient should first be interviewed for their health history. Choice *B* is incorrect, as the medical record is not always accurate; this information should be verified with the patient. Choice *C* and *D* may be consulted after attempts to obtain information from the patient. In cases where the patient is a poor historian or unable to answer questions, family, friends, or caregivers may be appropriate to garner patient information from.

45. D: The answer is Choice *D*. In total patient care, each nurse is assigned a group of patients by the charge nurse. The assignments vary between shifts, with less focus on continuity. Functional nursing occurs when the charge nurse delegates tasks. Primary care nursing features one nurse taking responsibility for a patient's overall plan of care throughout their stay, and team nursing is characterized by a group of nurses delivering patient care.

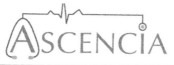

46. A: Choice *A* is correct, as it describes the barrier in accessing electronic health records that requires reverting to the historical methods of obtaining records, such as email, fax, and mail, which are slower. Choices *B*, *C*, and *D* are incorrect, as these describe the benefits of having electronic health records that are interoperable, usable, and conducive to widespread availability.

47. D: The correct answer is Choice *D* as picture boards or electronic touch screens with shapes or words are powerful tools to augment communication with a patient who has hearing impairments. Choice *A* is inappropriate because it is the patient's preference for whether to wear hearing aids or not. Choice *B* may not improve the patient's reception of voice depending on the type of hearing loss and may be interpreted as aggression. Choice *C* may make the patient feel uncomfortable and may not facilitate improved hearing or understanding.

48. D: Choice *D* is correct as it can accommodate increased learning opportunities for both visually impaired and blind patients. Choice *A* is incorrect because it assumes that the patient requires an escort. Choice *B* is incorrect; braille on signs is invaluable to blind patients who may expect that they will have wayfinding via braille on signs indicating clinical office numbers, elevators, restrooms, and other common places within a healthcare organization. Choice *C* is incorrect as the healthcare organization is expected to provide this service in the same manner that foreign language interpretation is accommodated.

49. D: The answer is Choice *D*, as the hospital command center is the designated centralized location where most communication will occur.

50. C: Within a Nursing Professional Practice Model, core values like compassion and advocacy serve as the ethical foundation for nursing practice. These values significantly impact interactions with both patients and colleagues, fostering a culture of respect, trust, and collaboration. Choice *A* is incorrect because the core values within a Nursing Professional Practice Model are primarily focused on ethical principles rather than administrative principles or management efficiency. Choice *B* is incorrect because the core values do not primarily revolve around efficiency and timeliness. Choice *D* is incorrect because the core values do not emphasize cost-effectiveness or resource allocation.

51. D: Choice *D* is correct; it is an intervention that can occur in the immediate time frame, and the family has been consulted and agrees upon it. Choice *A* is incorrect as it restricts the family's access to the patient. Choice *B* is incorrect as it is insensitive and does not provide support or comfort to the family in the moment. Choice *C* is incorrect as it does not provide coping strategies for the family currently; however, it is a good resource for preparing for coping after a patient passes.

52. D: Choice *D* is correct, as a handoff report must be completed covering at the least the patient's history, assessment, medications, and review of the plan of care. Choice *A* is incorrect, as just punching in does not mean that the responsibility of care for the patient has started. Choice *B* is incorrect, as the plan of care should be revised by the oncoming shift to ensure it is based on the most recent assessment and vital signs. Choice *C* is incorrect, as it is not reasonable to have the interdisciplinary team meet for every transfer of care. A patient may have multiple levels of care and different providers involved through the continuum.

53. A: The answer is Choice *A*. A learning needs assessment measures an existing gap between the current practice and anticipated practice. In this instance, the nurse educator will perform a learning needs assessment to determine the level of education required for nasogastric tubes. This can be done through a survey, observation, discussions with the nurses, safety report information, and other methods.

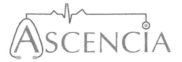

54. B: The correct answer is Choice *B*. The priority is to use the Confusion Assessment Method (CAM) to assess whether the patient has disorganized thinking, which gives an indication of delirium. The nurse would also review the medical record to identify any cognitive changes from the last shift, make sure the alarm is on, and notify the physician. Benzodiazepine can cause patients to be more relaxed but can also worsen agitation. Performing an assessment by using the CAM takes precedence.

55. B: The answer is Choice *B*, as giving patient medication is the responsibility of the direct care staff. The charge nurse is responsible for coordinating the unit flow, being aware of the competence of staff so that tasks can be effectively delegated, providing customer service, and restocking supplies and equipment.

56. D: Choice *D* is correct, as structural measures include factors such as patient-to-provider ratios, board certification among employed care providers, and electronic record safety features adopted. Choice *A* is incorrect, as this is related to the methods used to enhance health outcomes. Choice *B* is incorrect; this measure looks at the rates of achieved results and consequences due to receiving care. Choice *C* is incorrect, as this is not one of the quality outcome measures.

57. D: Choice *D* is correct; the CDC advocates for incorporating vegetarian protein sources in addition to lean meats. Choice *A* is incorrect as low-fat milk and milk products are promoted as part of a healthy diet. Choice *C* is incorrect; vegetables that are in a wide range of colors provide increased nutrition. Choice *D* is incorrect; lean meats, shellfish, and poultry may be healthy additions.

58. A: The correct answer is Choice *A*, as the patient should always be provided with the opportunity to participate in using a translation service to facilitate communication. Choice *B* is not correct, as the niece is a minor. This should only be considered if the patient is clinically unstable and there is no other option. Choice *C* is not the best choice as other healthcare providers should only be relied on to translate if they have received professional training to serve as a healthcare translator. Choice *D* is incorrect as the patient nodding may not reflect understanding and continuing to communicate in this manner would be detrimental to patient care.

59. A: The correct choice is Choice *A*. Assisting the patient with ambulation is an immediate fall risk prevention strategy and also provides the longer-term benefit of allowing the patient to ambulate in attempts to prevent deconditioning and even atrophy. The patient does not have any problems with her cognition, so she would not need to be placed close to the nurse's station, have frequent checks, or have a bed alarm in place (note the importance of educating this patient on using the call light). *Note that some facilities recognize bed alarms as a restraint, so the nurse must be aware of organizational policies and procedures.

60. D: Choice *D* is correct as severe dehydration due to fluid loss, electrolyte shifts, and lack of homeostasis in temperature control can induce seizures. Choices *A*, *B*, and *C* are incorrect as they are symptoms of mild to moderate dehydration, not severe.

61. C: The correct answer is Choice *C* as summarizing is a method used to show a message was received and acknowledged. Using reflection to mirror feelings builds trust with patients. Choice *A* is incorrect because questions should be open-ended to prevent leading and gain more information. Choice *B* is incorrect as a public space may have distractions and excessive noise. The patient should be provided an area that is free from interruptions and private so that the patient feels comfortable discussing vulnerable concerns. Choice *D* is incorrect as using devices during conversation can be seen as not being interested or not listening. This will detract from the goal of using active listening to improve communication with patients.

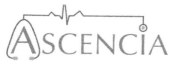

62. A: Choice *A* is correct, as the fundamental basis for patient-centered care is understanding and anticipating the needs of the patient to incorporate their preferences, needs, and values into their care. This is accomplished through the establishment of respectful communication and trust. Choice *B* is incorrect, as resources and the patient's potential constraints and barriers should be anticipated for all patient populations. Choice *C* is incorrect, as patient-centered care through the continuum expands beyond the inpatient setting. Choice *D* is incorrect, as needed resources must be anticipated and identified prior to discharge to prevent issues from occurring.

63. D: The correct answer is Choice *D*. A postoperative ileus is defined as a lack of intestinal motility. The other options also describe an ileus, as well as other conditions like constipation.

64. B: The answer is Choice *B*. All the choices are cause for concern regarding nursing retention. However, the priority would be the injuries directly caused by vacating staff. High turnover can lead to medical error and patient harm.

65. B: The correct answer is Choice *B*, as printed out downtime forms that the staff is familiar with should always be accessible and available in the working unit for nursing staff. When a downtime is scheduled, these forms should be distributed in advance. Choice *A* is not appropriate because the patient record should be kept up to date without gaps in the clinical care that is provided. Choice *C* does not provide a standardized method of documentation, which is an evidence-based best practice. Choice *D* is not a reasonable option because patients are not required to be relocated to another unit for a downtime procedure.

66. B: Adverse events like medication errors or nosocomial infections can have broader consequences, including increased costs, reputation damage to the healthcare facility, and compromised patient safety. Reporting is essential for prompt mitigation of these effects. Choice *A* is incorrect because it inaccurately suggests that adverse events have minimal impact on healthcare facilities and misrepresents reporting as primarily a legal requirement. Choice *C* is incorrect because it oversimplifies the consequences of adverse events, implying that they result in staff retraining and portraying reporting as a routine administrative process. Choice *D* is incorrect because it falsely asserts that adverse events solely affect the immediate patient and do not have broader impacts on healthcare facilities, which is not reflective of the actual consequences.

67. B: The correct answer is Choice *B* because Situation, not Status, is a part of the SBAR communication tool. Choices *A*, *C*, and *D* are incorrect as they are all a part of the SBAR communication tool.

68. D: Choice *D* is correct as basing hiring only on the candidate's years of experience excludes candidates that may represent a positive change to traditional values and will increase the pool of selection for leadership that has a broader cultural representation. Choice *B* is incorrect; a diverse community is a reason that bicultural representation in leadership is needed to promote justice and inclusivity. Choices *A* and *C* are both methods that leadership may use to improve cultural competence in staff but do not create diversity within leadership.

69. B: The correct answer is Choice *B*. When a peripherally inserted central catheter (PICC) is inserted, the environment is contained in an attempt to maintain asepsis. The door is kept closed and extra visitors and staff are limited. Maximum barrier precautions should be maintained, which includes sterile gloves, sterile gown, sterile drape, and mask. The site is typically prepared with a >0.5 percent chlorhexidine solution (exceptions are typically related to allergies).

70. A: The correct answer is Choice *A*. The nurse can implement all of the measures except administering medications to the patient that can worsen delirium. Temazepam is a benzodiazepine,

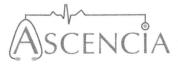

which has an adverse effect of change in the level of consciousness. Sleep is, however, important for the patient with delirium. Sleep-promoting measures include adopting a bedtime routine.

71. C: Choice *C* is correct, as education should begin at the onset of discussion to provide the patient with the information needed to obtain informed consent and initiate learning to assist the patient with control over their own care if the treatment is opted for. Choices *A*, *B*, and *D* are incorrect, as the patient requires education prior to the treatment beginning to fully understand the risks versus benefits as well as to determine if it is manageable post-hospitalization.

72. A: The answer is Choice *A*. All the options are important components of conflict management. However, the need for the nursing team to work together to deliver effective quality of care to the patient would most correspond with safe delivery of care. Safety is the priority in the work environment because conflict can cause harm to the patient.

73. A: Continuity, within the "5 C's" framework, highlights the significance of sustaining ongoing, consistent relationships between patients and their healthcare providers. This contributes to a positive and personalized patient experience. Choice *B* is incorrect because consistency refers to providing reliable care and communication. Choice *C* is incorrect because coordination emphasizes effective collaboration among healthcare providers and departments. Choice *D* is incorrect because caring underscores the importance of empathy and compassion in patient-centered care.

74. B: The correct answer is Choice *B*. The next step on the analgesic ladder would be a weak opioid, such as codeine or hydrocodone. The steps are a nonopioid analgesic, a weak opioid analgesic, a strong opioid, and then non-pharmacological invasive or minimally invasive treatments. An adjuvant, such as amitriptyline or gabapentin, may also be administered with any step.

75. C: Choice *C* is correct, as the patient should be assessed for appropriateness of transitional care within a rehabilitative facility to further recover prior to returning to the home environment. Choice *A* is incorrect, as the nurse should not ignore the concerns of the wife. Other options should be explored. Choice *B* is incorrect because it may provide a brief episode of respite for the spouse but will not provide assistance with activities of daily care on a 24/7 basis. Choice *D* is incorrect, as the patient will likely have restrictions, and this is not conducive to providing a healing environment for the patient.

76. B: The correct choice is Choice *B*. The nurse maintains the patient's body temperature with a warm blanket. A low core body temperature both pre- and postoperatively could be a contributing factor to a surgical site infection. Providing warmth to the patient postoperatively can help reduce the consequences of hypothermia. The initial wound dressing should never be removed without either the medical provider or surgeon's orders. Continuous monitoring of the integumentary status would not be indicated for early detection of an SSI. Routine assessment of generalized skin integrity, along with scheduled wound dressing changes are important. The use of incentive spirometry decreases the risk of pneumonia.

77. D: The correct answer is Choice *D*; while this pain rating tool was originally created to assess pain in young children unable to verbalize their feelings, it has been found to be invaluable to assess pain through all age ranges. Choices *A*, *B*, and *C* are incorrect because they do not encompass all age ranges that the tool may be useful to.

78. B: The correct answer is Choice *B* as the patient is not in acute distress; however, there is potential that this could be a known adverse effect to the vancomycin or an allergic reaction. Requesting guidance and consultation from the rapid response team to evaluate the patient is the most appropriate action in this case. Choice *A* is not the best choice as the patient is not in respiratory or cardiovascular arrest.

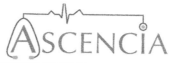

Choice C is incorrect as the attending nurse should not leave a patient who is in real or potential distress. Choice D is incorrect as the patient has exhibited symptoms that indicate decompensation in clinical status and must be addressed immediately to identify the cause.

79. A: The correct answer is Choice A. Using the teach-back technique, the patient can receive education from the nurse and explain what she learned using her own words. The nurse evaluates the patient's understanding of the content and does not quiz her knowledge. Teach-back uses open-ended questions instead of yes/no questions. Additionally, teach-back is not typically time-consuming.

80. B: The answer is Choice B, as a patient with a closed fracture is classified as non-urgent. An urgent patient has an open fracture or large wound. An emergent patient has a life-threatening injury, such as a trauma. The term *wounded* is not part of the classification.

81. C: The execution phase is where the project plan is put into practical action. It is the phase where project tasks are carried out, and the project progresses toward its objectives. Choice A is the phase where the project is formally initiated, and the project's purpose and initial constraints are defined. Choice B is the phase where project objectives, scope, schedule, budget, and resource requirements are detailed, setting the foundation for the execution phase. Choice D is a phase that runs concurrently with execution and involves oversight and control of project activities but is not primarily focused on the practical implementation of the project plan.

82. C: The correct answer is Choice C as the Assessment should include the patient's status, interventions completed, current patient status, and the nurse's judgment of the underlying cause of the deteriorating health condition. Choice A is incorrect as the medical history would be communicated in the Background. Choices B and D are both incorrect as these components would be communicated during the Recommendations.

83. B: Choice B is correct as it has been reported that incorporating spiritual and cultural preferences in care can positively affect the patient's decision-making process. Choice A is incorrect as compliance is not increased with guilt, and incorporating spiritual preferences can lessen patient distress. Choices C and D are incorrect as promoting the patient's spiritual preferences can decrease anxiety and depression while improving quality of life.

84. D: The correct answer is Choice D. The common complications of the PICC line are central line-associated bloodstream infection (CLABSI), venous thromboembolism (VTE), and mechanical failure. Central venous catheter (CVC) insertions can cause a pneumothorax due to the anatomical position to the clavicle and rib, such as the subclavian vein.

85. B: The correct choice is Choice B. A healthy work environment is one that has available personal protective equipment to protect from transmission of pathogens, voluntary overtime to provide adequate staffing, proper sharps disposal to protect from injury, and training available for the proper transferring techniques of patients. Additionally, a healthy work environment does not tolerate bullying or lateral violence.

86. D: The answer is Choice D. In this step, the ability to change is demonstrated through pilot trials when the opportunity for adjustments can be addressed. The awareness phase involves creating awareness among staff. In the desire stage, a desire is created among staff for the change. Next, knowledge is provided through education.

87. B: Choice B is correct as a comprehensive, multi-modal approach that includes pharmacological and alternative pain-relieving methods can have a synergistic effect on pain relief.

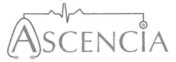

88. A: The correct answer is Choice *A*; a major barrier to completing sufficient hand-offs is time restrictions as a nurse often must provide a hand-off of two to six patients to, at times, multiple nurses. Choice *B* is incorrect as standardized checklists are encouraged to promote compliance and consistency. Choice *C* is incorrect as patients (and their families at the patient's approval) are encouraged to participate in patient-centered hand-offs. Choice *D* is incorrect as HIPAA standards provide guidelines to keep patient information confidential and within the healthcare team that requires it to provide patient care.

89. A: Choice *A* is correct, as the nurse should first consider the patient's preferred style of learning in order to create education that will be succinct and effective. Choice *B* is incorrect, as educational degrees do not always indicate the patient's learning style or level of ability to understand complex ideas. Choices *C* and *D* are important considerations that should be assessed to create patient-centered education that can be delivered within the time allotted; however, the preferred style of learning should be the priority.

90. A: Choice *A* is correct as implicit or subconscious bias may be either positive or negative beliefs and assumptions. Choices *B*, *C*, and *D* are incorrect as they are all characteristics of subconscious bias.

91. A: The correct answer is Choice *A*. Malignant hyperthermia causes an extreme release of calcium by the skeletal muscle cells when the patient is exposed to anesthetic drugs due to a genetic trait. The hypermetabolic state leads to muscle rigidity and can compromise vital organs.

92. D: Choice *D* is correct, as the name and contact information of the referred service provider should be provided to the patient prior to discharge, as well as the first scheduled appointment, if available. Choice *A* is incorrect; the patient may be provided with the options available for outpatient care services, but the nurse should not offer an opinion of one service provider being superior to another. Choice *B* is incorrect; the patient should contact their insurance company directly for the costs of treatment. Choice *C* is incorrect; if possible, the nurse should attempt to have services and a first appointment set up with the patient's preferred choice of outpatient provider prior to discharge.

93. C: Choice *C* is correct as the form must be completed, signed by the patient, and notarized in order to be legally binding. Choice *A* is not correct as it does not require an attorney's signature. Choice *B* is not correct as this form is not required to be filed with a courthouse; however, completed copies should be provided to the patient's primary healthcare provider and facility where care is occurring. Choice *D* is incorrect; while it is encouraged that the patient notifies the healthcare proxy and discusses wishes, this is not essential to completing an advance directive.

94. D: The answer is Choice *D*. Reflective practice is being mindful of a situation, analyzing the events that occurred, and contemplating on nursing actions. As a result, the nurse increases his knowledge base and skills. Clinical reasoning is a systematic approach to decision-making. Professional empowerment describes the nurse's autonomy and independent practice. Professional engagement refers to the motivation and involvement of the nurse.

95. A: The correct answer is Choice *A*; closed-loop communication is a tool that employs a process to determine that the message is delivered clearly and succinctly, confirms reception from the receiver, and affirmatively verifies for accuracy. Choices *B*, *C*, and *D* are all communication techniques that support that the receiver has received a message but do not endorse the closed-loop confirmation that the message received is the message that was intended.

96. A: Choice *A* is the correct answer as a risk assessment is a tool used to proactively identify potential gaps in care and analyze the effects that this deficit may cause. Choice *B* is incorrect because it would

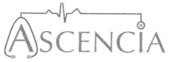

obtain qualitative data on the patient's perception of care but would not identify risks that are process issues. Choices C and D are incorrect because these will elicit staff and provider views and experiences but will not help identify the root causes of the cultural and linguistic needs of the organization.

97. C: The correct answer is Choice C. One purpose of the safety huddle is to share safety concerns from the previous shift in anticipation of issues before they arise. This can help foster a culture of awareness of any identified problems. The purpose is not to solve problems, invite upper management, or thoroughly review safety concerns from last week. A safety huddle is supposed to be brief with open communication from the frontline staff.

98. B: The correct answer is Choice B. To prevent postoperative pneumonia, the patient should be mobilized and ambulated in the hallway. Other pneumonia prevention measures are encouraging deep breathing and coughing, using an incentive spirometer, performing oral care, and having the patient sit in the chair. The patient would not be given acetaminophen for a temperature of less than 101°F/ 38.3°C. A wound culture would not be ordered unless the wound had signs of infection. The nurse should reassess the patient's vital signs, but this would not be the first action.

99. A: Choice A, a standardized report form, is the most effective way to ensure that pertinent information relating to the patient's ongoing care is relayed. This will facilitate the report from the EMS staff transporting the patient to the receiving staff. Choice B is incorrect; it would be unsafe and negligent, as the patient's family and caregivers may not be able to provide a health history, and they may not have the knowledge or medical expertise to relay the full clinical details necessary in a handoff. Choice C is incorrect, as this would include information that would not be related to the patient's current hospitalization events. Choice D is a part of the report but would not constitute a complete handoff.

100. A: The answer is Choice A. The chief nursing officer (CNO) advises how orientation can be structured to meet the nursing strategic plan and organizational goals. The nurse manager and director of nursing would be responsible for the needs of specific nursing units. Although the CNO provides input and suggestions on new policies and procedures, they would not create all the policies and procedures for the nursing unit.

101. D: The correct answer is Choice D as informational presentations, such as an administrative forum to provide organizational updates, are a type of formal communication. Choices A, B, and C are all considered informal types of communication.

102. C: Choice C is correct as not sharing the same native language has been shown to cause a significant rift in patient-provider communication. Choice A may have an influence on patient-provider communication; however, solely on its own, it is incorrect because there is a higher risk listed. Poor healthcare communication can further disproportion disadvantaged group, Choice B, but disadvantaged groups are not a communication barrier. Choice D is incorrect as an age gap between patient and provider is less detrimental to the patient relationship than not accommodating for preferred language.

103. A: The correct choice is Choice A. Evidence-based practice promotes a standardized approach to nursing care that incorporates scientific-based outcomes to guide decisions in support of excellent patient outcomes. A Root Cause Analysis (RCA) is a quality improvement method that seeks to identify the root cause of an issue when there is harm or breakdown in care. Failure Mode and Effects Analysis (FMEA) analyzes events or problems of potential harm before it occurs. Lean healthcare minimizes waste and eliminates items that do not provide value to patient care.

Answer Explanations #2

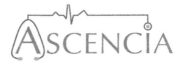

104. C: The correct answer is Choice C. Patients who need to void should be in a normal position to promote bladder emptying. The other options are not the best choice. The patient should walk to the toilet instead of using a bedpan whenever possible. A bladder scanner may be used once the patient voids. An epidural can cause urinary retention, but because the patient needs to void, the response should indicate an intervention or action.

105. C: Choice C is correct, as high readmission rates result in decreases of financial incentives from insurance companies and Medicaid/Medicare reimbursement rates. Choices A, B, and D are incorrect; per reported patient survey data, high admission rates result in lower patient satisfaction, poor patient outcomes, and a lack of trust from the community.

106. D: The answer is Choice D. The nurse manager is using a transformational leadership style. This type of style focuses on a greater vision, inspires employees to work toward a goal, and aims for high-quality patient outcomes. The other leadership styles do not apply. A democratic leader asks for staff input to make decisions. The servant leader is focused on meeting the individual needs of the employee. The transactional leader operates by managing tasks and expecting compliance.

107. C: The correct answer is Choice C as forms of explicit bias include racist comments, favoritism in granting work advancements, unfair pay, and sexual harassment. Choices A and D are incorrect as implicit bias may be positive or negative and tends to guide decisions and outcomes. Choice B is incorrect; it is implicit bias that is unconscious and unrealized. Explicit bias is described as overt and known.

108. C: The answer is Choice C. The emergency plan must be organized to respond to a worst-case scenario and avoid chaos. However, emergencies can be unpredictable, and the plan equips the staff for how to best respond. The exact steps that will happen cannot be predicted.

109. C: The correct answer is Choice C. The nurse plays the important role of reviewing the medication list and clarifying any discrepancies with the healthcare provider. The patient normally takes a multivitamin at home that will need to be brought to the provider's attention if it is not ordered on admission. The other options are not a priority. The pharmacist is collecting the medication data and would likely note the last medication doses. Teach-back education is often provided for new medications and medications that will be ordered upon discharge. Ordering the most cost-effective medication would also occur on discharge.

110. A: Choice A is correct as less than 3000 milligrams of sodium per day is recommended for individuals with mild cardiac disease. Choice B is incorrect as this amount is too high and would be recommended for healthy individuals. Choice C is incorrect; less than 2000 milligrams is recommended for individuals with moderate to severe heart failure. Choice D is incorrect as this amount is severely restrictive and should not be followed unless monitored by a healthcare provider.

111. D: Choice D is correct as this would be the patient's next of kin based on the choices available. Choices A, B, and C all have ethical concerns.

112. B: The answer is Choice B. The preparedness phase involves planning for the disaster and activation of the emergency plan. Mock drills are performed to identify gaps in practice. During the mitigation phase, community risks are assessed. The response phase is initiated when the emergency occurs, and the recovery phase is the return to a stable state.

113. C: The correct answer is Choice C. The patient's behavior may show unmet needs, including the need to be toileted, eat or drink, or walk. Physical and chemical restraints should be reserved for the patient who is at risk for harming themselves or others. Both physical and chemical restraints can make

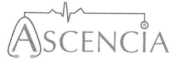

this specific patient WORSE. Lastly, assisting the patient back to bed most likely will not address the root issue and the patient will likely get right back out of bed again.

114. B: The correct answer is Choice *B*. After performing hand hygiene, donning the appropriate personal protective equipment (PPE), and scrubbing the port access site with chlorhexidine, the nurse palpates the port with the nondominant gloved hand. Next, the nurse stabilizes the port body, inserts the non-coring needle perpendicular to the port body, and flushes the port.

115. B: The answer is Choice *B*. A shared governance council is a collaboration among nursing staff and leaders to make decisions within the organization. These councils give a voice to the staff nurse and empower nurses to provide high-quality care.

116. C: Choice *C* is the correct choice; a communication board that covers essential and common patient requests and needs will facilitate a more comprehensive understanding between the patient and the nurse. Choice *A* is not the best answer as this may have too many choices that are not relevant to immediate needs and would not be useful for a patient who has a visual impairment. Choice *B* is not correct because communication boards should be easy to understand with simple concepts that are unlikely to be misconstrued by the audience. Choice *D* is incorrect as this may place stress on the patient and discourage use.

117. C: Choice *C* is correct, as the patient should be given time to get used to the tracheostomy care and slowly given education and tasks that they are comfortable doing in the beginning of the learning process. Choice *A* is incorrect; forcing the patient to do things that they are not comfortable doing is harmful to the nurse/patient relationship and does not promote patient-centered care. Choice *B* is incorrect, the nurse may include the patient's family and caregiver, but the patient will also need to learn and feel comfortable with the care routine prior to discharge. Choice *D* is incorrect because the patient must be able to demonstrate the ability to care for the new tracheostomy tube to be safe for discharge.

118. B: The correct answer is Choice *B*. The nurse first inspects the external catheter for any obvious kinks or clamped lumens. Next, the nurse helps the patient to reposition. If the lumen is still occluded, the nurse instills a low-dose fibrinolytic agent. An occluded lumen should never be ignored because the patient is at risk for further complications, including infection.

119. A: The answer is Choice *A*. Retention is often related to recognition, workload, competitive wages, available resources, opportunities of growth, and financial benefits.

120. B: Choice *B* is correct as consistent aerobic activity (thirty minutes per day for five days per week) increases cardiovascular strength, promotes euglycemia, and stabilizes weight. Choice *A* is incorrect; this caloric intake is not sufficient for an adult and does not improve cardiac function. Choice *C* is incorrect as this interval is not enough to provide results. A dietician, Choice *D*, may assist in controlling weight and preventing diabetes but does not increase vascular strength.

121. B: Choice *B* is correct as a limited code allows the patient to choose the life-saving interventions that they prefer. Choice *A* is incorrect as the patient wants a specific life-saving intervention. DNR status would allow for natural death. Choice *C* is incorrect as this provides all life-saving interventions, including being intubated and defibrillated—which the patient chose not to elect for. Choice *D* is incorrect as a health crisis and emergency can happen at any time regardless of age or health. It is standard practice for code status to be addressed by the provider with each patient encounter. If a code status is not listed, the care team assumes full code.

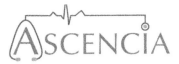

122. B: The correct answer is Choice *B*. A mock downtime drill is important because patients are at risk for a medication error when staff do not have access to the electronic record. The goal for the drill is to ensure that staff are aware of downtime procedures to reduce patient harm. Knowing the location of emergency equipment, storage of excess equipment, and observation of stairwells are not part of a mock downtime drill.

123. C: The answer is Choice *C*. The strategic plan is an organizational strategy that supports decision-making to steer the organization towards goals, and it often involves the mission and vision of the institution. An assessment of organizational strengths and weaknesses is part of a SWOT analysis that identifies strengths, weaknesses, opportunities for growth, and threats. This could be a method used for strategic planning. An inspired vision that the manager models for his staff is a characteristic of transformational leadership. A statement that describes how the organization will provide care to the community is the organizational vision.

124. A: The correct answer is Choice *A*. If medication reconciliation is not performed properly, the patient is at risk for readmission. The other options are not correct. The patient's pharmacy will maintain a list of medications prescribed for that pharmacy, but there may be missing medications if the patient uses more than one pharmacy, over-the-counter medications, or supplements. The physician is actively involved with medication reconciliation to determine whether the patient's home medications are necessary during the hospital admission. The pharmacist will document prescribed medications, over-the-counter drugs, vitamins, and supplements.

125. D: The correct choice is Choice *D*. Because transitions in care can create an opportunity of risk to patient safety, teach-back is an effective method to ascertain that the patient understands his discharge instructions. Providing detailed instructions to the ambulance driver about the patient's new medication will not guarantee that the patient understands once he is home. Explaining about the pulmonologist appointment will not ensure that the patient follows up. More effectively, the nurse could make the appointment for the patient. Discharge planning should start at admission, not when the patient is leaving.

Dear Medical Surgical Nurse test taker,

Great job completing this study guide. The hard work and effort you put into your test preparation will help you succeed on your upcoming Medical Surgical Nurse exam. Thank you for letting us be a part of your education journey!

We have other study guides and products that you may find useful. Search for us on Amazon.com or let us know what you are looking for. We offer a wide variety of study guides that cover a multitude of subjects.

If you would like to share your success stories with us, or if you have a suggestion, comment, or concern, please send us an email at support@triviumtestprep.com.

Thanks again for choosing us!
Happy Testing
Ascencia

Made in the USA
Middletown, DE
06 December 2024

66278792R00110